IMPROVING URBAN ENVIRONMENTS

Strategies for Healthier and More Sustainable Cities

IMPROVING URBAN ENVIRONMENTS

Strategies for Healthier and More Sustainable Cities

Edited by

Marco Ragazzi, PhD

APPLE ACADEMIC PRESS

Apple Academic Press Inc.
3333 Mistwell Crescent
Oakville, ON L6L 0A2
Canada

Apple Academic Press Inc.
9 Spinnaker Way
Waretown, NJ 08758
USA

Exclusive worldwide distribution by CRC Press, a member of Taylor & Francis Group

No claim to original U.S. Government works

Printed in the United States of America on acid-free paper

International Standard Book Number-13: 978-1-77188-416-7 (Hardcover)

International Standard Book Number-13: 978-1-77188-417-4 (eBook)

Library and Archives Canada Cataloguing in Publication

Improving urban environments : strategies for healthier and more sustainable cities / edited by Marco Ragazzi, PhD.

Includes bibliographical references and index.
Issued in print and electronic formats.
ISBN 978-1-77188-416-7 (hardcover).--ISBN 978-1-77188-417-4 (pdf)
1. Urban health. 2. Sustainable urban development. 3. Sustainable living. I. Ragazzi, Marco, author, editor

RA566.7.I46 2016 362.1'042 C2016-900183-0 C2016-900184-9

Library of Congress Cataloging-in-Publication Data

Names: Ragazzi, Marco, editor.
Title: Improving urban environments : strategies for healthier and more sustainable cities / edited by Marco Ragazzi, PhD.
Description: Oakville, ON ; Waretown, NJ : Apple Academic Press, 2016. |
Includes bibliographical references and index.
Identifiers: LCCN 2016000479 (print) | LCCN 2016010002 (ebook) | ISBN 9781771884167 (hardcover : alk. paper) | ISBN 9781771884174 (eBook) | ISBN 9781771884174 ()
Subjects: LCSH: Municipal engineering. | City planning--Environmental aspects. | Urban ecology (Sociology) | Environmental protection. | Sustainable urban development.
Classification: LCC TD159 .I47 2016 (print) | LCC TD159 (ebook) | DDC 628--dc23
LC record available at http://lccn.loc.gov/2016000479

Apple Academic Press also publishes its books in a variety of electronic formats. Some content that appears in print may not be available in electronic format. For information about Apple Academic Press products, visit our website at **www.appleacademicpress.com** and the CRC Press website at **www.crcpress.com**

About the Editor

MARCO RAGAZZI

Marco Ragazzi has a PhD in sanitary engineering from Milan Polytechnic, Italy. The author or co-author of more than 500 publications (111 in the Scopus database), he is currently a member of the Department of Civil, Environmental, and Mechanical Engineering at the University of Trento, Italy. His research interests include solid waste and wastewater management, environmental engineering, and environmental impact risk assessment.

Contents

Acknowledgment and How to Cite

The editor and publisher thank each of the authors who contributed to this book. The chapters in this book were previously published elsewhere. To cite the work contained in this book and to view the individual permissions, please refer to the citation at the beginning of each chapter. Each chapter was carefully selected by the editor; the result is a book that looks at healthy and sustainable cities. The chapters included are broken into six sections, which describe the following topics:

- Chapter 1 gives us a good overview of the many strategies that contribute to a healthy urban environment, from indoor air quality and urban heat island mitigation to sustainable transportation, urban densification, carbon foot printing and several others. The authors summarize 16 research articles and conclude with take-away messages and emerging future research needs.
- In chapter 2, we point out the latest practical and sustainable strategies for particulate matter reduction, which has become a necessity for the future of human and environmental health.
- In chapter 3, we offer an inventory of emissions from different sources in order to find the sources that are most significant, followed by some strategies to reduce emissions, from both environmental and economic points of view.
- The authors of chapter 4 use a case study to assess how new transit systems will be able to help cities reduce transportation impacts on air quality.
- The principle of photocatalytic concrete is elaborated in chapter 5, followed by a description of past research indicating important influencing factors for the purifying process.
- The study in chapter 6 revealed that using solely engineering solutions for solid-waste management is not sufficient.
- In chapter 7, the research results help define the optimal mechanical pretreatment in order to achieve the optimal balance between green house gas emissions and heat-and-power production.
- The authors of chapter 8 examine in depth the changes that need to take place in order to induce water management companies to improve their systems and local authorities to update their urban planning and building regulations, while organizing effective information campaigns that will

encourage end users to look for more efficient technologies in plumbing, building, sanitation, and others.

- The authors of chapter 9 developed and optimized a novel vertical membrane bioreactor to reduce the problems of pollutant removal from wastewater and the volume of produced sludge from a bench-scale to field-scale systems.
- In chapter 10, the authors advocate energy benchmarking of commercial buildings in order to give the market greater incentive to seek out superior energy performance.
- Chapter 11 presents an energy pattern analysis of a waste water treatment plant, creating a methodological framework by which other such studies can be replicated to generate data with respect to various scales of treatment and choice of treatment technology.
- Chapter 12 offers an overall systems approach that includes perspectives on different sub-systems and technologies.
- The final article, chapter 13, provides a framework for multi-scale urban ecosystem health assessment and its applications in management from global, national, regional and local viewpoints.

List of Contributors

Tiberiu Apostol
Dept. of Energy Production and Use, Politehnica, University of Bucharest, Romania

Adrian Badea
Prof., Department of Energy Production and Use, University Politehnica of Bucharest

Anne Beeldens
Belgian Road Research Center (BRRC), Woluwedal 42, 1200 Brussels, Belgium

Andrea Bolognesi
Department of Civil, Chemical, Environmental and Materials Engineering (DICAM), University of Bologna (Alma Mater), Viale Risorgimento 2; Bologna 40136, Italy

Elia Boonen
Belgian Road Research Center (BRRC), Woluwedal 42, 1200 Brussels, Belgium

Cristiana Bragalli
Department of Civil, Chemical, Environmental and Materials Engineering (DICAM), University of Bologna (Alma Mater), Viale Risorgimento 2; Bologna 40136, Italy

Sara Branchini
Centro Antartide, Via Rizzoli 3, Bologna 40125, Italy

Marilyn A Brown
School of Public Policy, Georgia Institute of Technology, D M Smith Building, 685 Cherry Street, Room 312, Atlanta, GA 30332-0345, USA

Cynthia Carliell-Marquet
Department of Civil Engineering, University of Birmingham, Birmingham, UK

So-Ryong Chae
Department of Biomedical, Chemical and Environmental Engineering, 701 Engineering Research Center, University of Cincinnati, Cincinnati, OH

Bin Chen
State Key Joint Laboratory of Environment Simulation and Pollution Control, School of Environment, Beijing Normal University, Beijing 100875, China

Mikhail Chester
Civil, Environmental, and Sustainability Engineering, School of Sustainability, Arizona State University, 501 E Tyler Mall Room 252, Mail Code 5306, Tempe, AZ 86287-5306, USA

Jin-Ho Chung
Daewoo Institute of Construction Technology, Gyeonggi-do 440-200, Korea

Giulio Conte
Ambiente Italia S.r.l., Via Carlo Poerio 39, Milano 20129, Italy

Sabrina Copelli
Department of Science and High Technology, University of Insubria, Italy

Matt Cox
School of Public Policy, Georgia Institute of Technology, D M Smith Building, 685 Cherry Street, Room 312, Atlanta, GA 30332-0345, USA

Alessandro De Carli
Department of Economic Sciences, University of Udine, Via Palladio 8, Udine 33100, Italy

William Eisenstein
Center for Resource Efficient Communities, University of California, Berkeley, 390 Wurster Hall #1839, Berkeley, CA 94720, USA

Zoe Elizabeth
Institute of the Environment and Sustainability, California Center for Sustainable Communities, University of California, Los Angeles, LaKretz Hall, Suite 300, 619 Charles E Young Dr. East, Los Angeles, CA 90095-1496, USA

Renuka Gurusinghe
Department of Civil Engineering, Faculty of Engineering Technology, The Open University of Sri Lanka, Nawala, Nugegoda, Sri Lanka.

Jukka Heinonen
University of Iceland, Faculty of Civil and Environmental Engineering, Iceland

Yong-Rok Heo
Daewoo Institute of Construction Technology, Gyeonggi-do 440-200, Korea

Sunil Herat
Griffith School of Engineering, Nathan Campus, Griffith University, Queensland, Australia.

Arpad Horvath
University of California Berkeley, Department of Civil and Environmental Engineering, USA

Gabriela Ionescu
Dept. of Energy Production and Use, Politehnica University of Bucharest, Romania,

Seppo Junnila
Aalto University, Department of Real Estate, Planning and Geoinformatics, Finland

Seok-Tae Kang
Department of Civil Engineering, Kyung Hee University, Gyeonggi-do 446-701, Korea

Arun Kansal
Department of Natural Resources, TERI University, 10 Institutional Area, Vasant Kunj, New Delhi, India

Joong-Won Lee
Department of Architecture, Sungkyunkwan University, 2066 Seobu-ro Jangan-gu, Suwon-si, Gyeonggi-do 440-746, Korea

Sang-Min Lee
Department of Environmental Engineering, Kongju National University, Chungcheongnam-do 330-717, Korea

Tae-Goo Lee
Department of Architecture, Semyung University, 65 Semyung-ro, Jecheonsi, Chungbuk 390-711, Korea

Chiara Lenzi
Department of Civil, Chemical, Environmental and Materials Engineering (DICAM), University of Bologna (Alma Mater), Viale Risorgimento 2; Bologna 40136, Italy

Bandunee Champika Liyanage
Department of Civil Engineering, Faculty of Engineering Technology, The Open University of Sri Lanka, Nawala, Nugegoda, Sri Lanka.

Gengyuan Liu
State Key Joint Laboratory of Environment Simulation and Pollution Control, School of Environment, Beijing Normal University, Beijing 100875, China

Fabio Masi
IRIDRA S.r.l., Via La Marmora, 51, Firenze 50121, Italy

Salvatore Masi
School of Engineering, University of Basilicata, Viale dell'Ateneo Lucano 10, Potenza I-85100, Italy

Antonio Massarutto
Department of Economic Sciences, University of Udine, Via Palladio 8, Udine 33100, Italy

Juan Matute
Luskin School of Public Affairs, Local Climate Change Initiative, University of California, Los Angeles, Box 165606, 3250 Public Affairs Building, Los Angeles, CA 90095-1656, USA

Stephanie Pincetl
Institute of the Environment and Sustainability, California Center for Sustainable Communities, University of California, Los Angeles, LaKretz Hall, Suite 300, 619 Charles E Young Dr. East, Los Angeles, CA 90095-1496, USA

Marco Pollastri
Centro Antartide, Via Rizzoli 3, Bologna 40125, Italy

Ilaria Principi
Ambiente Italia S.r.l., Via Carlo Poerio 39, Milano 20129, Italy

Massimo Raboni
Department of Science and High Technology, University of Insubria, Italy

Elena Cristina Rada
Dept. of Civil Environmental and Mechanical Engineering, University of Trento, Italy

Marco Ragazzi
Dept. of Civil, Environmental and Mechanical Engineering, University of Trento, Trento, Italy

Thorsten Schuetze
Department of Architecture, Sungkyunkwan University, 2066 Seobu-ro Jangan-gu, Suwon-si, Gyeonggi-do 440-746, Korea

Hang-Sik Shin
Department of Civil and Environmental Engineering, Korea Advanced Institute of Science & Technology, Daejeon 305-701, Korea

Pratima Singh
Department of Energy and Environment, TERI University, New Delhi, India

Meirong Su
State Key Joint Laboratory of Environment Simulation and Pollution Control, School of Environment, Beijing Normal University, Beijing 100875, China

Xiaojing Sun
School of Public Policy, Georgia Institute of Technology, D M Smith Building, 685 Cherry Street, Room 312, Atlanta, GA 30332-0345, USA

Masafumi Tateda
Department of Environmental Engineering, Toyama Prefectural University, Toyama, Japan.

Vincenzo Torretta
Dept. of Science and High Technology, University of Insubria, Italy

Ettore Trulli
School of Engineering, University of Basilicata, Viale dell'Ateneo Lucano 10, Potenza I-85100, Italy

Linyu Xu
State Key Joint Laboratory of Environment Simulation and Pollution Control, School of Environment, Beijing Normal University, Beijing 100875, China

Zhifeng Yang
State Key Joint Laboratory of Environment Simulation and Pollution Control, School of Environment, Beijing Normal University, Beijing 100875, China
\

M. Zandonai
ALPI BIOGAS – Competence Center for Biogas, Bolzano, 39100, Italy

Yanwei Zhao
State Key Joint Laboratory of Environment Simulation and Pollution Control, School of Environment, Beijing Normal University, Beijing 100875, China

Lixiao Zhang
State Key Joint Laboratory of Environment Simulation and Pollution Control, School of Environment, Beijing Normal University, Beijing 100875, China

Yan Zhang
State Key Joint Laboratory of Environment Simulation and Pollution Control, School of Environment, Beijing Normal University, Beijing 100875, China

Introduction

Cities are complex systems, which means that creating sustainable urban environments is a challenging goal. No single strategy—or even several strategies—will be enough to achieve healthy urban environments. We must look at elements as varied as urban air quality, inner-city transportation infrastructure, municipal waste management, building construction, municipal water management, and overall energy consumption. Each of these must then be examined from the perspectives of sustainability and health. We must determine which strategies within each topic will contribute most to our ultimate goal—healthy, sustainable cities.

The chapters within this book were chosen to lead city planners, policymakers, and researchers further down the road that will take us toward tomorrow's sustainable urban environments. Each chapter offers specific steps in that process.

—Marco Ragazzi, PhD

Environmental assessments have been developed with increasing emphasis since the wide-scale emergence of environmental concerns in the 1970s. However, after decades there is still plenty of room left for development. These assessments are also rapidly becoming more and more crucial as we seem to be reaching the boundaries of the carrying capacity of our planet. Assessments of the emissions from the built environment and especially of the interactions between human communities and emissions are in a very central role in the quest to solve the great problem of sustainable living. Policymakers and professionals in various fields urgently need reliable data on the current conditions and realistic future projections, as well as robust and scientifically defensible models for decision making. This recognition was the main motivation to call for Chapter 1. This editorial provides brief summaries and discussions on the 16 articles of a Focus Issue, depicting the several interesting perspectives they offer to advance the state of the art. The authors encourage academics, practitioners, government, industry, individual consumers, and other decision makers to utilize the available findings and develop the domain of environmental assessment of the built environment further. Indeed, the authors hope that the Focus Issue is merely a kernel of a significantly large future body of literature.

Chapter 2 presents an overview of practical strategies that can be adopted for reducing the particulate matter concentration in urban areas. Each strategy is analyzed taking into account the latest results of the scientific literature. A discussion useful for pointing out some problems to be solved for their correct adoptions completes the paper.

Chapter 3 describes the particulate matter pollution in a Northern Italian city: Varese. The city is distinguished by a particular orographic and meteorological situation, characterized by valleys and heavy rainfalls. Nevertheless the urban area is interested by particulate matter pollution mainly due to heating systems and traffic. Here some corrective strategies in order to reduce PM air pollution have been presented, applied and evaluated by the means of a simplified model which considers emissions and meteorological conditions.

Public transportation systems are often part of strategies to reduce urban environmental impacts from passenger transportation, yet comprehensive energy and environmental life-cycle measures, including upfront infrastructure effects and indirect and supply chain processes, are rarely considered. Using the new bus rapid transit and light rail lines in Los Angeles, near-term and long-term life-cycle impact assessments are developed in Chapter 4, including consideration of reduced automobile travel. Energy consumption and emissions of greenhouse gases and criteria pollutants are assessed, as well the potential for smog and respiratory impacts. Results show that life-cycle infrastructure, vehicle, and energy production components significantly increase the footprint of each mode (by 48–100% for energy and greenhouse gases, and up to 6200% for environmental impacts), and emerging technologies and renewable electricity standards will significantly reduce impacts. Life-cycle results are identified as either local (in Los Angeles) or remote, and show how the decision to build and operate a transit system in a city produces environmental impacts far outside of geopolitical boundaries. Ensuring shifts of between

20–30% of transit riders from automobiles will result in passenger transportation greenhouse gas reductions for the city, and the larger the shift, the quicker the payback, which should be considered for time-specific environmental goals.

Photocatalytic concrete constitutes a promising technique to reduce a number of air contaminants such as NO_x and VOC's, especially at sites with a high level of pollution: highly trafficked canyon streets, road tunnels, the urban environment, etc. Ideally, the photocatalyst, titanium dioxide, is introduced in the top layer of the concrete pavement for best results. In addition, the combination of TiO_2 with cement-based products offers some synergistic advantages, as the reaction products can be adsorbed at the surface and subsequently be washed away by rain. A first application has been studied by the Belgian Road Research Center (BRRC) on the side roads of a main entrance axis in Antwerp with the installation of 10.000 m^2 of photocatalytic concrete paving blocks. For now however, the translation of laboratory testing towards results in situ remains critical of demonstrating the effectiveness in large scale applications. Moreover, the durability of the air cleaning characteristic with time remains challenging for application in concrete roads. From this perspective, several new trial applications have been initiated in Belgium in recent years to assess the "real life" behavior, including a field site set up in the Leopold II tunnel of Brussels and the construction of new photocatalytic pavements on industrial zones in the cities of Wijnegem and Lier (province of Antwerp). Chapter 5 first gives a short overview of the photocatalytic principle applied in concrete, to continue with some main results of the laboratory research recognizing the important parameters that come into play. In addition, some of the methods and results, obtained for the existing application in Antwerp (2005) and during the implementation of the new realizations in Wijnegem and Lier (2010–2012) and in Brussels (2011–2013), will be presented.

The case study in chapter 6 investigates better and sustainable waste management for a given area in Sri Lanka. A questionnaire and field surveys were performed in a small local authority adjacent to Colombo, the capital city. Composting for organic waste and incineration for non-compostable waste were found to be important treatment methods for solid-waste management. The reduction of solid waste is a critical process for sustainable management. Currently, people in the area do not have much interest in waste recycling to decrease the cost of solid-waste management. It was therefore concluded that raising people's awareness would play an important role in the reduction of solid waste. A suitable waste-management plan needs to be made for each community and area. The situation and conditions of every area is different, therefore each community needs to make an effort to find its own better and sustainable solid-waste management process.

The planning actions in municipal solid waste (MSW) management must follow strategies aimed at obtaining economies of scale. At the regional basin, a proper feasibility analysis of treatment and disposal plants should be based on the collection and analysis of data available on production rate and technological characteristics of waste. Considering the regulations constraint, the energy recovery is limited by the creation of small or medium-sized incineration plants, while separated collection strongly influences the heating value of the residual MSW. Moreover, separated collection of organic fraction in non-densely populated area is burdensome and difficult to manage. Chapter 7 shows the results of the analysis carried out to evaluate the potential energy recovery using a combined cycle for the incineration of mechanically pre-treated MSW in Basilicata, a non-densely populated region in Southern Italy. In order to focalize the role of sieving as pre-treatment, the evaluation on the MSW sieved fraction heating value was presented. Co-generative (heat and power production) plant was compared to other MSW management solutions (e.g., direct landfilling), also considering the environmental impact in terms of greenhouse gases (GHGs) emissions.

The excessive use of water is damaging European groundwater and rivers: their environmental conditions are often below the "good status" that—according to Water Framework Directive 2000/60—should be reached by 2015. The already critical situation is tending to get worse because of climate change. Even in water rich countries, urban wastewater is still one of the main sources of water pollution. Currently, urban soil sealing and "conventional" rainwater management, which were planned to quickly move rainwater away from roofs and streets, are increasing the flood risk. "Green" technologies and approaches would permit a reduction in water abstraction and wastewater production while improving urban hydrological response to heavy rains. In Chapter 8, the Life+ WATACLIC project has been implemented to promote such sustainable technologies and approaches in Italy, however the results show huge difficulties: apparently water saving and sustainable urban water management have only low interest amongst the general public and even with public administrations and the relevant industrial sectors. In such a cultural and technical context, the project is bringing a new point of view to public debate. In the long term, the project will certainly have a positive impact, but most likely it will require more time than initially expected.

In nutrient-sensitive estuaries, wastewater treatment plants (WWTPs) are required to implement more advanced treatment methods in order to meet increasingly stringent effluent guidelines for organic matter and nutrients. To comply with current and anticipated water quality regulations and to reduce the volume of produced sludge, the athors of Chapter 9 successfully developed a vertical membrane bioreactor (VMBR) that is composed of anoxic (lower layer) and oxic (upper layer) zones in one reactor. Since 2009, the VMBR has been commercialized (Q = 1100–16,000 m3/d) under the trade-name of DMBR™ for recycling of municipal wastewater in South Korea. In this study, the authors explore the performance and stability of the full-scale systems. As a result, it was found that the DMBR™ systems showed excellent removal efficiencies of organic substances, suspended solids (SS) and *Escherichia coli* (*E. coli*). Moreover, average removal efficiencies of total nitrogen (TN) and total phosphorus (TP) by the DMBR™ systems were found to be 79% and 90% at 18 °C, 8.3 h HRT and 41 d SRT. Moreover, transmembrane pressure (TMP) was maintained below 40 kPa at a flux of 18 $L/m^2/h$ (LMH) more than 300 days. Average specific energy consumption of the full-scale DMBR™ systems was found to be 0.94 kWh/m^3.

US cities are beginning to experiment with a regulatory approach to address information failures in the real estate market by mandating the energy benchmarking of commercial buildings. Understanding how a commercial building uses energy has many benefits; for example, it helps building owners and tenants identify poor-performing buildings and subsystems and it enables high-performing buildings to achieve greater occupancy rates, rents, and property values. Chapter 10 estimates the possible impacts of a national energy benchmarking mandate through analysis chiefly utilizing the Georgia Tech version of the National Energy Modeling System (GT-NEMS). Correcting input discount rates results in a 4.0% reduction in projected energy consumption for seven major classes of equipment relative to the reference case forecast in 2020, rising to 8.7% in 2035. Thus, the official US energy forecasts appear to overestimate future energy consumption by underestimating investments in energy-efficient equipment. Further discount rate reductions spurred by benchmarking policies yield another 1.3–1.4% in energy savings in 2020, increasing to 2.2–2.4% in 2035. Benchmarking would increase the purchase of energy-efficient equipment, reducing energy bills, CO_2 emissions, and conventional air pollution. Achieving comparable CO_2 savings would require more than tripling existing US solar capacity. Our analysis suggests that nearly 90% of the energy saved by a national benchmarking policy would benefit metropolitan areas, and the policy's benefits would outweigh its costs, both to the private sector and society broadly.

Various forms of energy are used during a wastewater treatment process like electrical, manual, fuel, chemical etc. Most of the earlier studies have focused only on electrical energy intensity of large-scale centralized wastewater treatment plants (WWTPs). Chapter 11 presents a methodological framework for analysing manual, mechanical, chemical and electrical energy consumption in a small-scaled WWTP. The methodology has been demonstrated on a small-scale WWTP in an institutional area. Total energy intensity of the plant is 1.046 kWh/m^3 of wastewater treated. Electrical energy is only about half of the total energy consumption. Manual energy also has a significant share, which means that the small-scale treat- ment plants offer significant employment opportunities in newly industrializing countries and replaces fossil fuel-based energy with renewable. There is a lack of sufficient data in the literature for comparison, and few studies have reported values that vary significantly due to the difference in scale, scope of the study and the choice of the treatment technologies. Replication of similar studies and generation of data in this area will offer directions for decision on choice of the scale of wastewater treatment process from the considerations of energy and climate change mitigation strategies.

The construction and service of urban infrastructure systems and buildings involves immense resource consumption. Cities are responsible for the largest component of global energy, water, and food consumption as well as related sewage and organic waste production. Due to ongoing global urbanization, in which the largest sector of the global population lives in cities which are already built, global level strategies need to be developed that facilitate both the sustainable construction of new cities and the re-development of existing urban environments. A very promising approach in this regard is the decentralization and building integration of environmentally sound infrastructure systems for integrated resource management. Chapter 12 discusses such new and innovative building services engineering systems, which could contribute to increased energy efficiency, resource productivity, and urban resilience. Applied research and development projects in Germany, which are based on integrated system approaches for the integrated and environmentally sound management of energy, water and organic waste, are used as examples. The findings are especially promising and can be used to stimulate further research and development, including economical aspects which are crucial for sustainable urban (re-)development.

Urban ecosystem health assessments can be applied extensively in urban management to evaluate the status quo of the urban ecosystem, identify the limiting factors, identify key problems, optimize the scheme and guide ecological regulation. Regarding the multi-layer roles of urban ecosystems, urban ecosystem health should be assessed at different scales with each assessment providing a specific reference to urban management from its own viewpoint. Therefore, a novel framework of multi-scale urban ecosystem health assessment is established on global, national, regional and local scales in Chapter 13. A demonstration of the framework is shown by using a case study in Guangzhou City, China, where urban ecosystem health assessment is conducted in the order of global, national, regional, and local scales, from macro to micro, and rough to detailed analysis. The new multi-scale framework can be utilized to generate a more comprehensive understanding of urban ecosystem health, more accurate orientation of urban development, and more feasible regulation and management programs when compared with the traditional urban ecosystem health assessment focusing at the local scale.

PART I

OVERVIEW

CHAPTER 1

Environmental Assessments in the Built Environment: Crucial yet Underdeveloped

JUKKA HEINONEN, ARPAD HORVATH, AND SEPPO JUNNILA

1.1 INTRODUCTION

Creating sustainable human settlements will be one of the grand challenges in the coming decades (Rees and Wackernagel 1996, Glaeser 2011, Seto et al 2014). On a global scale we overuse our planet's renewable capacity (WWF 2014), and we seem to have already crossed the planetary boundaries regarding several impact categories and in others the limits are getting closer (Rockström et al 2009). It is vital to investigate what would make cities sustainable in order to fulfil our ever increasing needs and find opportunities to live, work, urbanize in a more environmentally affordable way.

However, we currently seem to be much more capable of measuring and describing the problems than finding solutions. For example, the confidence in anthropogenic greenhouse gases (GHGs) causing the climate change is very high (Cook et al 2013), and in that urban areas cause the majority of the emissions (Seto et al 2014), but very different views exist regarding the relationship between the urban structure and GHG emissions. Traditionally higher density has been connected to lower emissions (e.g. Kenworthy 2006, Brown et al 2009, Glaeser and Kahn 2010) and thus it has become the dominant urban development target around the developed countries. Notwithstanding, an increasing number of studies have indicated that density might not be a sufficient indicator for GHGs (Jones and Kammen 2013, Minx et al 2013, Baur et al 2014), and that higher density might even drive higher emissions (Heinonen et al 2011, Wiedenhofer et al 2013). Regarding many other impact categories the situation is very similar. Higher density is tied to reduced private driving, which decreases the particulate matter emissions, but the intake fractions have been shown to increase at the same time, potentially more than enough to compen- sate the reductions in the emissions (Apte et al 2012). Furthermore, balancing the assessments between the emissions occurring now and those taking place in the future is an issue where two different, but widely used and accepted, assessment approaches can lead to very different outcomes and policy implications (e.g. Schwietzke et al 2011, Säynäjoki et al 2012).

Assessments of the emissions and especially of the interactions between human communities and emissions are thus in a very central role in the quest to solve the problem of sustainable living. This, combined with all the contradictions and shortcomings in the current environmental assessment practices, gave motivation for this focus issue, and led us to invite especially papers based on empirical and quantitative data. At the closure of the issue we cannot say that the sustainability problem would be solved, far from that as recent evidence shows (Seto et al 2014, WWF 2014), but the collection of published papers certainly forms an interesting combination of perspectives on the big issues and advances the state of the art by one step.

Altogether 15 research papers and one perspective were accepted for this focus issue during 2012–2014. The issues concerned in the papers vary from indoor air quality and urban heat island (UHI) mitigation to (more) sustainable transportation, urban densification, carbon footprinting and several others. In the next sections we shortly summarize the perspectives offered by these studies and the suggestions they give to advance the quest for sustainable living. In the final section, we discuss the overall take-away messages and the existing and emerging future research needs.

1.2 PERSPECTIVES ON AND IMPROVEMENTS TO ENVIRONMENTAL ASSESSMENTS IN THE BUILT ENVIRONMENT

1.2.1 IMPROVING TRANSPORTATION ASSESSMENTS

Reducing private driving and increasing the share of public transport has established a strong position in the environmental sustainability strategies from country to local community levels. The issue rose to a significant role in this Focus Issue as well, especially from the perspective of how infrastructure should be taken into account in environmental burden assessments. In two letters the authors stress that despite the strong position of transportation in general, the impacts of the transportation infrastructure development have been undermined in this branch of research (Chester et al 2013, Thorne et al 2014). Eckelman (2013) discusses in his perspective further the issues presented by Chester et al. Strongly related to the previous, Gosse and Clarens (2013) discuss utility and the currently weak position of systems thinking in the optimization of urban roadway design, arguing that success in the efforts to reduce the traffic-related costs and emissions require systems thinking over the whole life cycle.

Chester et al (2013) point out that the infrastructure impacts can be significant and variable across different impact categories in comparison to the use phase emissions, with decades-long payback times at worst. They notice that the assessment results are highly sensitive to the assumed modal shifts as the result of investing into improving public transit sys- tems. While assessing the life-cycle emissions, Chester et al separate the locally occurring from those caused elsewhere. In his perspective, Eckelman discusses how in transportation decision-making one problem is the spreading of environmental burdens far outside the local community responsible for the transportation infrastructure. He stresses the importance of separating the local emissions and those occurring elsewhere in future assessments, as done by Chester et al. He also gives credit to Chester et al for using consequential life-cycle assessment (LCA) to demonstrate the tem- poral perspective of the caused environmental burdens and the potential future gains, and raises the issue as an important direction of assessment development.

Thorne et al (2014) approach the infrastructure issue from a different perspective. They demonstrate the applicability of a regional advance mitigation planning (RAMP) framework in assessing the ecosystem impacts of infrastructure development. Using the San Francisco Bay Area in California as a case, they show how a regional integrated assessment of multiple projects brings advantages when compared to traditional project-by-project assessments. An integrated assessment framework like RAMP could enable such planning which would prevent infrastructure development from cutting the habitat reserves into a myriad of insufficiently small land pieces. Additional interest should evoke the thought that combined mitigation solutions might reduce the required land acquisitions and thus the transaction costs.

Gosse and Clarens apply LCA on the infrastructure system level to analyze how a modal shift to bicycling affects the costs and emissions of transportation. Continuing in similar vein to the previously-described letters, the authors stress the importance of a system- wide scope and life-cycle perspective in assessing the environmental burdens from transportation. They show that turning parking space into bike lanes can reduce time and environmental burdens, and require only minimal investments, if done so that increased bicycling does not delay traffic.

While the three papers are very different in nature, their common quality is that they all stress the importance of comprehensive assessments with wider scopes than traditionally adopted. An analogous consequence is that the assessments become very complex and include a lot of uncertainty. However, it is easy to justify a conclusion that more and more comprehensive assessments are mandatory to assist the policy-making processes in finding the best-available options.

1.2.2 UNDERSTANDING THE NEGATIVE HEALTH IMPACTS OF THE BUILT ENVIRONMENT

Nazaroff (2013) presents an overview on how climate change will or might affect indoor air quality and related health impacts. He argues that while the health consequences of different indoor and outdoor emissions have been studied relatively extensively, little attention has been paid so far to the effect of climate change on these. He concludes that the impact of climate change is very complex and that the net impact is difficult to assess. On one hand, there are certain benefits that the presumed shift away from fossil fuels in both power generation and in transportation will bring to indoor air quality. On the other, the endeavor for higher building energy efficiency might show in decreased ventilation levels and cause the concentrations of indoor-sourced emissions to increase. In addition, climate change itself will lead to changes in the existence and harmfulness of certain natural causes of negative health impacts, such as windblown dust.

From the assessment perspective, Nazaroff's paper raises again the problem of high complexity of comprehensive assessments in the context of the built environment. A very high level of uncertainty has to be accepted especially when looking into the future, with changes both in the natural environment and in the built environment affecting the assessments concurrently. Nazaroff also mentions the interesting yet not always recognized paradox of the built environment, namely that even if emissions decrease, human exposures might still increase. Apte et al (2012) give a good example of this by depicting how particulate matter exposures are higher in denser cities around the globe than in less urbanized areas, despite the well-documented decrease in transportation trip generation that typically comes with higher density.

1.2.3 UHI MEASUREMENT AND MITIGATION

Li et al (2013) approached UHI measurement and mitigation from the perspective of pavement materials, showing how higher permeability could offer a feasible way to significantly mitigate the surface and near-surface temperatures in urban settlements. They also show how permeable pavements can help in stormwater management. Li et al also argue that in the future assessments should reach wider life-cycle scopes. The direct impacts can already be measured with reasonable reliability, but life-cycle impacts of new technologies and materials are less known.

In their two-part contribution to this focus issue, Dan Li et al concentrate on another contribution to UHI mitigation, that of green and cool roofs. In the first part, Li and Bou-Zeid (2014) validate the simulation method and demonstrate how it reduces the temperature biases in comparison to several earlier simulation methods due to its ability to accommodate the variation in the intra-urban facets and the main hydrological processes. In the second part, Li et al (2014) employ the method in a simulation of the impacts of green and cool roof mitigation strategies on UHI in the Baltimore–Washington metropolitan area. They depict how both mitigation strategies show linear mitigation ability in optimal conditions (moisture/albedo). They suggest that the employed assessment method adds an important piece to UHI simulation via city-scale simulation, with sensitivity to heterogeneity in the intra-city canopies.

The UHI effect provides an example of a man-made environmental impact of which we have been aware for decades, but which still needs important development steps in environmental assessment and simulation techniques. The articles from Li et al (2013), Li and Bou-Zeid (2014) and Li et al (2014) are just such steps. However, both also stress the importance of further development needs in this area.

1.2.4 ANALYZING GHG EMISSIONS CAUSED BY DIFFERENT TYPES OF HUMAN SETTLEMENTS

As many as four letters in this Focus Issue are devoted to discussing GHG and to a lesser extent other emissions that human settlements cause by their users' and residents' consumption of goods and services. Heinonen et al (2013a, 2013b) assessed the carbon footprints of the residents of different types of human settlements in Finland and elaborate their analysis with time-use data to understand better the differences in the daily lives behind the varying carbon footprints. Minx et al (2013) look at the carbon footprints in the UK analyzing the impacts of the settlement type and several other variables. Goldstein et al (2013) enhance traditional urban metabolism (UM) analysis with LCA to form an UM approach capable of quantifying global environmental burdens. To nicely complement these four approaches, Ramaswami and Chavez (2013) present an analysis how different metrics should be used to understand the different perspectives of the energy and carbon intensities of cities.

Heinonen et al find in the first part of their study (2013a) that carbon footprints increase rather steadily with the income level from the least to the most urbanized, highest density areas in Finland. They analyze the lifestyles to understand the mechanisms behind the results, and with evidence from both monetary consumption data and time-use data they present a concept of parallel consumption as one explanation: how the reduced living spaces in the more urbanized areas are actually a trade-off with service spaces in near proximity, and how space consumption spreads outside the home even while homes are equipped to provide many of the searched services.

In the second part Heinonen et al restrict their analyses to the middle-income population and look at additional variables of housing type and motorization. The results depict interestingly how little impact these variables have on the overall carbon footprints when the same disposable income is given for each resident. With the same income, the apartment buildings are crowded with very small households and the economies-of-scale effect equalizes the carbon footprints. Regarding motorization, the cost of owning and operating a vehicle is so high that the non-motorized can spend significantly more on other consumption and thus reduce the positive impact of not driving.

Minx et al (2013) look at GHG emissions from two perspectives: from the more traditional territorially restricted and from consumption based. They show how the vast majority of the human settlements in the United Kingdom are importers of GHGs. In the territorial (scope 2) analysis, the level of urbanization seems to play a role in that GHG emissions increase towards the less urbanized areas, but when the consumption-based perspective is taken, the differences disappear almost completely. They also conclude, similarly to Heinonen et al that density is a poor indicator for carbon footprints, and that the emissions are much more strongly driven by socio-economic characteristics than density of a certain area.

There are several well-known problems related to carbon footprinting. In this Focus Issue, two author groups approach the issue using two different assessment methods or data sets, thus being able to analyze additional perspectives, especially the lifestyle differences explaining the findings. Both groups also call for more contributions, looking particularly at the lifestyles from various perspectives and advancing the assessments that way.

Goldstein et al (2013) on their part approach the issue from the opposite direction, utilizing LCA to enhance the traditional UM analysis. They call the approach UM-LCA and describe it as a third-generation UM framework. They show how the earlier-generation UM frameworks end up underestimating the actual environmental burdens due to their inability to properly capture the life-cycle impacts caused by a certain settlement. Their work aims clearly to enhance the UM methods, but as stated by the authors, the framework they propose is not ready, but is rather a first step in the right direction. They also propose an important further step, maybe the fourth-generation UM framework, in suggesting to bind the UM-LCA into the planetary boundaries approach presented some years ago by Rockström et al (2009).

As a kind of umbrella for all the above approaches, Ramaswami and Chavez (2013) discuss the best metric to describe the GHG or energy efficiency of a certain human settlement. They suggest that we should not even try to use a single metric, but actually understand the utility of different approaches and use them in the right way and in the right context. The regional energy and carbon intensity should be measured as an intensity relative to the gross domestic product, whereas the consumption-based assessment should use a per-capita basis. Their work could provide valuable guidance for policy makers seeking GHG mitigation strategies and grappling with highly variable assessment results coming from different sources.

1.2.5 DENSIFICATION PROSPECTS AND CONSEQUENCES

While the letters from Heinonen et al and Minx et al in this Focus Issue question the utility of densification as a vehicle to GHG mitigation, it remains a paradigm in urban planning policies in the developed countries due to the demonstrated connection to reducing private driving. In their letters, Brecheisen and Theis (2013) and Shmidt-Thomé et al (2013) concentrate on the issue of densification.

Schmidt-Thomé et al look at the prospects for densification using Soft-GIS data collected from Finland. Their hypothesis is that densification is a highly context-sensitive issue and thus perceived very differently in different locations. Giving some policy advice, the authors find that the residents tend to ex ante prefer the same degree of density in the future as they experience at the time of the interview. However, regarding large new residential development projects, the study found no correlation between the density of a development and the interest shown towards it. The authors conclude that densification development should be place-sensitive to understand the perceptions of the residents and target developments where they are received well.

From the perspective of this Focus Issue, Schmidt-Thomé et al suggest that context-sensitivity should be given more emphasis in planning and the type of Soft-GIS approach they employ could be the tool. Infill developments are not always perceived very well by the residents of a certain area, but by understanding the perceptions, better infill policies could be designed.

Schmidt-Thomé et al refrain from taking a stand on the environmental sustainability perspective of infill developments, while Brecheisen and Theis study the particular issue from a life-cycle energy requirements perspective. They employ LCA to study the energy requirements of a brownfield redevelopment project from the remediation until 10 years of use. Infill developments often require utilization of brownfield sites, creating a problematic situation since the remediation requirements may be significant. For Brecheisen and Theis the results are promising since the authors report the refurbished building to have reached nearly 50% lower use-phase energy consumption than the average in the area for the same building type, and the use-phase energy still dominates the life-cycle energy requirements after 10 years of use despite significant land removal and remediation requirements. Furthermore, the authors estimate that demolishing and constructing a new building would have tripled the energy requirements of the project.

1.2.6 ECONOMIC INCENTIVES

Mitigating the environmental harm caused by humans will require significant amount of capital if we are to achieve sustainable coexistence with nature. Yet it is much more likely that the improvement potentials will realize if there is economic incentive to invest in certain improvements. Cox et al (2013) and Gosse and Clarens (2013) approach their topics through the lens of economic and environmental feasibility.

Cox et al propose enhanced benchmarking for building energy efficiency, arguing that the current practices easily underestimate the savings potentials due to their weak recognition of future technological development. They find the efficiency improvements to be not just economically feasible, but also to reduce both criteria pollutants and GHG emissions. Furthermore, their analysis shows the benchmarking policies to economically benefit both the private sector and society. Gosse and Clarens' approach, as discussed in section 2.1, is very similar in that they also look for the opportunities to reduce life-cycle costs and show how it leads to reduced environmental burdens as well.

1.3 FINAL REMARKS

Environmental assessments have been developed since the wide-scale emergence of environmental concerns (mostly in rich countries) in the 1970s and even earlier. Still, after decades there is plenty of room left for further development. Environmental assessments are quickly becoming more and more crucial as we seem to be reaching the boundaries of the carrying capacity of our planet. Policy-makers and professionals in various fields urgently need reliable data on the current conditions and realistic future projections, as well as robust and scientifically defensible models for decision making.

This recognition was the main motivation to call for a Focus Issue on environmental assessment of the built environment. We can conclude that the published articles highlight and address the same point. Representing various fields and disciplines, a theme taken up in the majority of the letters is the requirement for further development in the assessment methods, while recognizing that important and crucial steps have been taken to improve environmental assessment techniques and analyses.

Now we hope academics, practitioners, government, industry, individual consumers, and other decision makers will get motivated to utilize the available findings and develop the domain of environmental assessment of the built environment further. Indeed, we hope that this Focus Issue is merely a kernel of a significantly large future body of literature.

REFERENCES

1. Apte J, Bombrun E and Marshall J 2012 Global intraurban intake fractions for primary air pollutants from vehicles and other distributed sources Environ. Sci. Technol. 46 3415–3423
2. Baur A, Thess M, Kleinschmit B and Creutzig F 2014 Urban climate change mitigation in Europe: looking at and beyond the role of population density J. Urban Plan. Dev. 140 1–12
3. Brecheisen T and Theis T 2013 The Chicago center for green technology: life-cycle assessment of a brownfield redevelopment project Environ. Res. Lett. 8 015038
4. Brown M, Southworth F and Sarzynski A 2009 The geography of metropolitan carbon footprints Policy Soc. 27 285–304
5. Chester M, Pincetl S, Eisenstein W and Matute J 2013 Infrastructure and automobile shifts: positioning transit to reduce life-cycle environmental impacts for urban sustainability goals Environ. Res. Lett. 8 015041
6. Cook J, Nuccitelli D, Green S, Richardson M, Winkler B, Painting R, Way R, Jacobs P and Skuce A 2013 Quantifying the consensus on anthropogenic global warming in the scientific literature Environ. Res. Lett. 8 024024
7. Cox M, Brown M and Sun X 2013 Energy benchmarking of commercial buildings: a low-cost pathway toward urban sustainability Environ. Res. Lett. 8 035018
8. Eckelman M 2013 Life cycle assessment in support of sustainable transportation Environ. Res. Lett. 8 021004
9. Glaeser E 2011 Cities, productivity, and quality of life Science 333 592–4
10. Glaeser E and Kahn M 2010 The greenness of cities: carbon dioxide emissions and urban development J. Urban Econ. 67 404–18
11. Goldstein B, Birkved M, Quitzau M-B and Hauschild M 2013 Quantification of urban metabolism through coupling with the life cycle assessment framework: concept development and case study Environ. Res. Lett. 8 035024
12. Gosse C and Clarens A 2013 Quantifying the total cost of infrastructure to enable environmentally preferable decisions: the case of urban roadway design Environ. Res. Lett. 8 015028
13. Heinonen J, Jalas M, Juntunen J, Ala-Mantila S and Junnila S 2013a Situated lifestyles: I. How lifestyles change along with the level of urbanization and what are the greenhouse gas implications, a study of Finland Environ. Res. Lett. 8 025003

14. Heinonen J, Jalas M, Juntunen J, Ala-Mantila S and Junnila S 2013b Situated lifestyles: II. The impacts of urban density, housing type and motorization on the greenhouse gas emissions of the middle income consumers in Finland Environ. Res. Lett. 8 035050
15. Heinonen J, Kyrö R and Junnila S 2011 Dense downtown living more carbon intense due to higher consumption: a case study of Helsinki Environ. Res. Lett. 6 034034
16. Jones C and Kammen D 2013 Spatial distribution of US Household carbon footprints reveals suburbanization undermines greenhouse gas benefits of urban population density Environ. Sci. Technol. 48 895–902
17. Kenworthy J 2006 The eco-city: ten key transport and planning dimensions for sustainable city development Environ. Urbanization 18 67–85
18. Li D and Bou-Zeid E 2014 Quality and sensitivity of high-resolution numerical simulation of urban heat islands Environ. Res. Lett. 9 055001
19. Li D, Bou-Zeid E and Oppenheimer M 2014 The effectiveness of cool and green roofs as urban heat island mitigation strategies Environ. Res. Lett. 9 055002
20. Li H, Harvey J, Holland T and Kayhanian M 2013 The use of reflective and permeable pavements as a potential practice for heat island mitigation and stormwater management Environ. Res. Lett. 8 015023
21. Minx J, Baiocchi G, Wiedmann T, Barrett J, Creutzig F, Feng K, Förster M, Pichler P, Weisz H and Hubacek K 2013 Carbon footprints of cities and other human settlements in the UK Environ. Res. Lett. 8 035039
22. Nazaroff W 2013 Exploring the consequences of climate change for indoor air quality Environ. Res. Lett. 8 015022
23. Ramaswami A and Chavez A 2013 What metrics best reflect the energy and carbon intensity of cities? Insights from theory and modeling of 20 US cities Environ. Res. Lett. 8 035011
24. Rees W and Wackernagel M 1996 Urban ecological footprints: why cities cannot be sustainable—and why they are a key to sustainability Environ. Impact Assses. Rev. 16 233–48
25. Rockström J et al 2009 A safe operating space for humanity Nature 461 472–5
26. Säynäjoki A, Heinonen J and Junnila S 2012 A scenario analysis of the life cycle greenhouse gas emissions of a new residential area Environ. Res. Lett. 7 034037
27. Schmidt-Thomé K, Haybatollahi M, Kyttä M and Korpi J 2013 The prospects for urban densification: a place-based study Environ. Res. Lett. 8 025020
28. Schwietzke S, Griffin M and Matthews S 2011 Relevance of emissions timing in biofuel greenhouse gases and climate impacts Environ. Sci. Technol. 45 8197–203
29. Seto K C et al 2014 Human settlements, infrastructure and spatial planning Climate Change 2014: Mitigation of Climate Change. Contribution of Working Group III to the 5th Assessment Report of the Intergovernmental Panel on Climate Change ed
30. O Edenhofer et al (Cambridge: Cambridge University Press) Thorne J, Huber P, O'Donoghue E and Santos M 2014 The use of regional advance mitigation planning (RAMP) to integrate transportation infrastructure impacts with sustainability; a perspective from the USA Environ. Res. Lett. 9 065001

31. Wiedenhofer D, Lenzen M and Steinberger J 2013 Energy requirements of consumption: urban form, climatic and socioeconomic factors, rebounds and their policy implications Energy Policy 63 696–707
32. WWF 2014 Living planet report 2014: species and spaces, people and places ed R McLellan, L Iyengar, B Jeffries and N Oerlemans (Gland, Switzerland: WWF)

PART II

IMPROVING URBAN AIR QUALITY

CHAPTER 2

Critical Analysis of Strategies for PM Reduction in Urban Areas

GABRIELA IONESCU, TIBERIU APOSTOL, ELENA CRISTINA RADA, MARCO RAGAZZI AND VINCENZO TORRETTA

2.1 INTRODUCTION

The globalization and rapid industrial development of urban cities has conducted to notable modifications on air quality. Environmental and social questions have been raised on air pollution. Among them, the particular matter (PM) may be the air pollutant that has the most commonly known environmental global effects. In the last two decades concerns on particulate matter concentration values in urban areas led to a number of researches on this type of pollutant [1,2]. According to Amato et al., [3] the atmospheric particulate matter (PM) is a complex mixture of components arising from a number of emission sources (anthropogenic, but also natural) and atmospheric processes (secondary PM) which have a variable diameter in the range 0.01 μm- 100 μm. The differences and amount of

PM is mainly influenced by complex interactions of the source characteristics with the geography, season and short-term meteorology of the site.

Depending on their aerodynamic diameter (ad), the PM is divided into three main categories:

- coarse fraction ranging from $2.5\mu m \leq a_d \leq 10\ \mu m$ is produced by mechanical processes such as erosion, grinding or suspension and may include marine aerosols, pollen and dust resulting from agricultural processes, roads etc..;
- fine fraction ranging from $0.1\ \mu m \leq a_d \leq 2.5\ \mu m$ is produced by means of clot particles ultrafine, or for heterogeneous nucleation;
- ultrafine fraction - $a_d \leq 0.1\ \mu m$ is produced by homogeneous nucleation vapor SO_2, NH_3, NO_x and products combustion which form new particles by condensation and grow for coagulation.

Measurements of fine particulate matter (PM_{10} and $PM_{2.5}$) have become an interest in air quality studies, mainly because they are associated with numerous health effects. Many epidemiological studies have demonstrated the toxicity of certain pollutants and the relationship between their emission and increased mortality and hospitalization [4,5]. Worldwide, about 3% of respiratory infection, 5% of cardiopulmonary and 8% of lung cancer deaths are attributed to PM exposure [6]. An investigation made in Arizona, where the $PM_{10\text{-}2.5}/PM_{10}$ average ratio is about 0.7, has observed associations between PM_{10}, $PM_{10\text{-}2.5}$ and total mortality [7]. The same association can be made with the study made in California (a desert region) suggesting a mortality effect of PM_{10} in a region where PM mass is dominated by coarse mode aerosols [8]. L. Perez et al., [9,10] have shown the association between significant levels of coarse PM resulted from human activity and daily mortality in Barcelona (Spain) and demonstrated the same effect of the particle from the Saharan dust. Over more, the cardiovascular and cerebrovascular mortality were associated with increased levels of coarse fractions (PM_1 and $PM_{2.5\text{–}10}$) [10]. It can be conclude that in dried-up regions the mortality increases on coarse PM presence.

In Europe the standards on ambient air quality and cleaner air is covered by Directive 2008/50/EC where the annul amount of $PM_{2.5}$ cannot exceed 25 $\mu g/m^3$ and 40 $\mu g/m^3$ for PM_{10} [11]. In 2013 the Environmental

Protection Agency (EPA) has lowered the allowable average concentration of certain PM with 20% respect to 2006 making it more drastic in comparison with the European standard. The new annual limit imposed for the $PM_{2.5}$ concentration is 12 μg/m^3 (primary) and 15 μg/m^3 (secondary), annual means, averaged over 3 years [12]. Recent studies in Europe have shown that PM_{10} levels increase from natural to kerbside sites. Especially in urban and kerbside stations, PM_{10} levels are above the EU annual PM_{10} standard for 2010 [14].

In the forthcoming years, the meteorological conditions and smoke events might increase due to the air pollution in relation with climate change. In this context the current paper points out the latest practical and sustainable strategies for PM reduction that have become a human health and environmental future necessity.

2.2 SOURCES OF PM EMISSIONS

The causes of air pollution episodes include various factors, e.g., emissions, local and synoptic-scale meteorological conditions, topography and atmospheric chemical processes [15,16,17]. The relative importance of such factors is dependent on the geographical region, its surrounding emission source areas and the related climatic characteristics, as well as the season of the year [18,19]. The produced PM can be divided in two main categories: primary (is the sum of the filterable and the condensable PM) and secondary PM (are particles that form through chemical reactions in the ambient air after dilution and condensation have occurred and generally belonged to the submicron $PM_{1.0}$ mode). Therefore the secondary PM formed include precursor such as Volatile Organic Compounds (VOC), ammonia, SO_2 and NO_x. In the emission inventory the secondary PM are not reported, only the precursor emissions.

Several studies have shown the mineral origin of PM_{10} and its silicates, carbonates, oxides and phosphates components which are more present in the $PM_{2.5-10}$ (coarse) fraction rather than in $PM_{2.5}$ (fine) particles [20,21,22]. Still, the mechanical abrasion of crustal materials which produces the amount $PM_{2.5}$ fraction may be notable to the ecosystem [23]. A study conducted in six urban sites from Europe revealed the major components in

$PM_{2.5}$ were carbonaceous compounds (POM+EC), secondary ions and SS, whereas those in $PM_{2.5\text{-}10}$ were soil derived compounds, carbonaceous compounds, SS and nitrate. All the measured and estimated components together accounted for 79–106% of $PM_{2.5}$ and 77–96% of PM $_{2.5\text{-}10}$ [24].

The primary PM is generated from industrial activities of fossil fuels in cogeneration plants, in diesel vehicles, in the residential sector but also from industrial processes in forms of $PM_{2.5}$ fines. The fine particles resulted from the fossil fuel combustion contain As, Be, Cd, Cr, Co, Pb, Mg, Ni, Zn and Se. The traffic-related source of PM concentration is given by road surface wear, tyre and brake wears. In 2005, Hueglin et al. studied trace elements from rural traffic sites and concluded that concentrations of Ba, Cu, Fe, Mo, Mn and Sb from brake wear traces gradually decrease from kerbside to urban background, near-city and rural sites [25]. Earlier studies reported an important concentration of Zn, Cd, Co, Cr, Cu, Hg, Mn, Mo, Ni, and Pb from tyre wear [26, 27].

The traffics related particles, which prevail on non-desert dust days, have more toxic effects than the ones originating from long-range transport, such as the Sahara dust.

Looking over the European situation, as compared to Central Europe, the urban areas of Southern Europe are sensibly more enriched in suspended PM_{10} mineral matter due to the intensive deposition of non-vehicular related dust on the pavement due to African dust outbreaks or construction/demolition may contribute decisively to supplement the mineral load over roads in Southern Europe. This difference is contribution to the PM levels of crustal components which can may be attributed largely to the higher dust accumulation and resuspension effect during dry conditions in the southern EU countries, whereas higher rainfall in the central EU countries may help to clean the road dust from streets [3].

Although few researches have been made on the particles resulted from small-scale combustion utilities (domestic boiler or small residential) [28], it is considered that these type emissions affect the PM load in the coarse $PM_{10-2.5}$ mode. The particle mass can be significantly influenced by the wind-blown soil and re-suspended street dust that are present also in the coarse particle fraction [29]. The $PM_{2.5}/PM_{10}$ ratios can varies from 0.4 up to 0.7 depending on site analyzed.

Taking into account the secondary particles, in Europe the annual PM_{10} and $PM_{2.5}$ concentrations are mainly affected by the regional aerosol background. As for chemical composition, Putaud et. al., demonstrated that organic matter appears more often as the major component of both PM_{10} and $PM_{2.5}$, with the exception of natural and rural background sites, where sulphate contribution appear to be much greater. As for chemical composition, the organic matter appears more often as the major component of both PM_{10} and $PM_{2.5}$, with the exception of natural and rural background sites, where sulphate contribution appear to be much greater [29].

The origins and sources of emission from long-range transport (LRT) and regional transport (RT) from local pollution (LP) could be distinguished. The Juda-Rezler et. al., reported, in Central Eastern European urban areas, that the high winter episodes of PM_{10} are for a large part caused by several anthropogenic emission processes that imply LRT, RT or LP sources, unfavorable synoptic-scale (anti-cyclonic circulation) and local meteorological conditions (very low temperature, low wind speeds, surface layer inversions) are also responsible for the occurrence of air pollution events [30]. The latter causes are completed by coal or wood combustion in cogeneration plants, but also the unfavorable winter (weather) conditions that increase the traffic emissions.

Due to the internal combustion engine, cars emit mostly fine and ultrafine particles. Aarnio et al., [31] and Niemi et al., [32] concluded that emissions from tyre and brake wear and also the resuspension of dust from the road surface as vehicular non-exhaust sources, represent one of the most important sources of air pollution at intersection sites. Note that if LP and RT sources are emitting a different level of PM concentrations, therefore the transboundary LRT particles can represent a source of episodic pollution caused by transnational PM migration. An investigation made in southern Finland pointed out the value of $PM_{2.5}$ is usually exceeded in this area due to LRT of pollutants from Eastern Europe. The study highlighted that the investigated LRT episodes were caused by emissions not only from open biomass burning, but emissions from ordinary anthropogenic sources (e.g. from energy production, traffic, industry and wood combustion) in Eastern Europe also cause significant episodes. It should be pointed out that emissions from agricultural waste burning and wildfires conduct to air pollution on large areas, especially in warm and dry periods of the year (late spring and summer) even at the distance over 1000 km from the fire areas [31,32].

In his latest work Srimuruganandam et. al., [14] presented the PM contribution in Chennai, India from diesel exhaust, gasoline exhaust, paved road dusts, brake lining dusts, brake pad dusts, marine aerosols and cooking exhausts. Results indicated that the emissions from diesel (PM_{10}= ~52%; $PM_{2.5}$= ~65%) and gasoline exhaust (PM_{10}= ~16%; $PM_{2.5}$= ~8%) vehicles are predominant sources at the study site. The emissions from cooking (PM_{10}=$PM_{2.5}$ = ~1.5%) and paved road dust (PM_{10}= $PM_{2.5}$= ~2.3%) are found to be low. Presence of marine aerosols and brake wear dusts in PM_{10} and $PM_{2.5}$ are found to be in trace quantities. Further modeling results demonstrated that diesel and gasoline emission contributions are also comparable with emission inventory results.

Another public transport source of air pollution is given by subway railway stations. High levels of particles have been found at subway and underground railway stations: the levels of PM_{10} and $PM_{2.5}$ at a subway station in Stockholm that were 5–10 times higher than on a busy street. It is estimated that the emission factors were found to be in the range 0.2–3 g $train^{-1}$ km^{-1} [33].

The combustion of coal for electricity and heat production contributes to the emissions of primary particles but also formation of secondary aerosols, from the derived reactions of sulphur dioxide (SO_2) and nitrogen oxides (NO_x) species to sulphate and nitrate. The critical period of air pollution is during winter, due to the long-lasting periods of high pressure, that are often accompanied by a state of thermal inversion that promote the accumulation of pollutants in the lower atmospheric layers. The amount and composition of the primary emissions are efficiently registered by various types of Air Pollution Emission Control Devices for Stationary Sources. Still the amount of emissions resulted from the local residential units or local activities remain under question due to the lack of accurate information.

Along with the burning of waste (as is [15, 34, 35, 36] or pre-treated [37, 15, 38, 39]) or primary fossil fuels, emissions associated with the extraction work quarries is a major source of particulate matter (aspects perceived also from the population [40]). The Life Cycle Assessment inventory can give an insight on the estimate amount of primary emissions by type of extraction. Still the lack of data inventory delays the implementation of a PM reduction strategy in this sector.

2.3 STRATEGIES FOR PM REDUCTION

The aim of the present research is to analyze a set of strategic solutions for the PM reduction without reducing the consumption of resources that plays a direct action (e.g., fuel substitution, the renewal of an automotive park, etc.) or limiting the energy consumption by acting indirectly (e.g. condensing boilers, solar panels, etc). The two strategies pose a long-term goal for which an assessment of the results can be made only after a few years of implementation.

An immediate possibility is represented by the removal of dust already present in the atmosphere (for example, through the washing of the roads) or the limits imposed during periods of criticality. In current investigations, the street sweeping combined with washing activities found a decrease of 7–10% and up to 24% in the ambient PM_{10} re-suspension from paved roads [41,42]. These measures are potentially easy to apply and their effectiveness is immediately evaluated. However Langston et al., [43] showed that the immediate effects on emissions reduction at urban areas where the number of the streets treated can be low. Amato et. al., suggests the street washing investigations on wider areas (some km2) in order to increase the absolute emission benefit.

It should be recognized that the pollutants involved are many; in fact, the contribution that the secondary particles on the total presence in the atmosphere is probably high, although studies are still in the investigation process.

Summarizing up the stationary power plants case the next measures for the particle emissions reduction are presented:

- rehabilitation of the present combustion wood plants and their transition on natural gas cogeneration sites.
- use of electrostatic precipitators for wood-fired applications are known already marketed for large systems, where the Swiss Fed-

eral Institute for Materials Testing, has successfully tested an electro cheap for fireplaces, wood stoves, pellets smaller than 30 kW, which reduces emissions from the combustion of wood 80 to 90% [28].

- retrofitting diesel and fuel oil.
- use of condensing boilers can improve the seasonal average efficiency of production and its applicable to all installations with fan. The temperature of exhaust gases from the traditional installations varies between 120°C and 140°C; lowering this value it is possible to recover about 1% of the low heating value for each 20°C reduction in temperature.
- use of solar panels are suggested by Taha, [44]: solar systems of up to 2 MW should be installed on the roofs of warehouses, parking lot structures, schools, and other commercial buildings throughout the state; solar energy projects of up to 20 MW in size should be built on public and private property.
- use of diesel fuel with low sulfur content – this simple strategy indicates the replace of fuel rich in sulfur with the low sulfur content as required by legislation thereby lowering the emission factor. Without reducing consumption the reduction of SO_x emissions can be significant.
- use of biodiesel in power plants is highly recommended not only for PM_{10} reduction but mostly for the inhibition of secondary reaction with gas precursors formation and in particular on SO_x.

In the transport case, the long term and seasonal measures proposed for PM reduction are:

- replacement of the heavy emitting aging vehicles- the abatement of transport emissions by renewing the vehicle park (Euro 5 for light duty vehicles, Euro 6 for heavy duty vehicles) is essential.
- replacement of diesel vehicles with natural gas or Liquid Petroleum Gas (LPG)- the main benefits of LPG are that it yields 50% less CO, 40% less HC, 35% less NO_x and has 50% less OFP (ozone forming potential) compared to gasoline. LPG is also free of particulates, the main pollutant of diesel and GDI engines [45].

- use of fuels with low sulfur content already impose by Directive 2003/17/EC with <50 ppm sulfur. Overmore biodiesel differs from petro-diesel due to its zero or ultralow natural sulphur content, it contains no aromatic or polyaromatic hydrocarbons, it has a higher cetane value, a lower heating value, better lubricity, higher viscosity, and a higher flash point.
- use of particulate filters on diesel engines can reduce more than 90% of the particulate emissions resulted.
- traffic alternate plates: the methods consist in blocking all vehicles bearing license plates with an even number on even days and odd-odd days. It is estimated that this measure, taken into consideration all the powers that are granted (buses, motorcycles, often commercial vehicles) might cause a reduction in the daily traffic of about 15% from the theoretical point of view.
- block traffic for the most heavy emitting aging vehicles- unlike alternate plates that measure is more focused as "hits" category of vehicles responsible for the majority of emissions from transport.
- speed moderation on the highway as strategy from PM reduction can be associate with the reduction of fuel consumption. In order to obtain concrete results, it must have an extension of time adequate. It does not seem a problem to apply a limit of 90 km/h for a few miles of highway) in winter period since the loss of time caused is very limited. The COPERT program correlates the emissions of CO_2, THC and CO for all vehicles. In earlier studies and simulations with COPERT program of the traffic flow and particle emissions produced it was observed a visible reduction of air pollution due to reduction of the speed mainly on highways. To this concern a recent innovative project on integrated monitoring by low cost sensors on the territory [46] has been proposed also for an enhanced management of the speed on an Italian highway.
- improvement of public transportation infrastructures and services (e.g. optimization of MSW collection system [47, 48]).

In the extraction work area, there might be the use of special spray to wet the area of the quarry and precipitate particles dispersed in the atmosphere during the work of extraction and transit of heavy vehicles in the area. In this sense there is not yet enough data to assess the actual effectiveness of this intervention: waiting for any new knowledge it was decided not to carry out calculations for this measure.

2.4 DISCUSSION AND DEVELOPMENTS

The choice of the PM reduction actions should be based on an 'appropriate technology concept' in terms of potential for prevention and reduction of PM, their applicability and their cost compared to the benefits brought in terms of emissions avoided.

On the contrary, typical situation decision makers have to face with concerns the absence of a quantification of the ratio cost-benefits for the area where they should activate an air quality action plan.

In reality, for most of the listed options the ratio Euro to be paid per kg of PM avoided can be assessed referring to the primary particulate. A similar ratio for secondary particulate is more difficult to be proposed as the reactions generating it are very complex.

An additional aspect to be taken into account is the presence of incentives that can affect the calculations: the difference between gross and net costs should be pointed out.

Moreover, a significant problem to be solved is the understanding of the viability of some actions: a limitation of the vehicle circulation has a reduced effect is no control is performed.

Other strategies show a high variability in results, as street washing.

The investigation of certain types of campaigns is logistically complex for researchers without the involvement of local authorities. To this concern in many European countries significant examples of collaboration among research institutions and administrative bodies (as environmental protection agencies) can be found also supported by EU funds.

REFERENCES

1. R. Vecchia, G. Marcazzana, G. Vallia, M. Ceriania, C. Antoniazzia, "The role of atmospheric dispersion in the seasonal variation of PM1and PM2.5 concentration and composition in the urban area of Milan (Italy)". Atmos. Environ., vol. 38, 2004, pp. 4437- 4446.
2. G. Hoek, B. Forsberg, M. Borowska, S. Hlawicza, E. Vaskovi, H. Welinder, M. Branis, I. Benes, F. Kotesovec, L.O. Hagen, J. Cyrys, M. Jantunen, W. Roemer, B. Brunekreef, "Wintertime PM10 and Black Smoke concentrations across Europe: results from the Peace study". Atmos. Environ., vol. 31, n. 21, 1997, pp. 3609–3622
3. [3]. F. Amato, X. Querol , C. Johansson, C. Nagl, A. Alastuey, "A review on the effectiveness of street sweeping, washing and dust suppressants as urban PM control methods". Sci. Total Environ., vol. 408, 2010, pp. 3070–3084.
4. H. Kan, R. Chena, S.Tong, "Ambient air pollution, climate change, and population health in China". Environ. Int., vol. 42, 2012, pp. 10–19.
5. A. Makria, N.s I. Stilianakisa, "Vulnerability to air pollution health effects", Int. J. Hyg. Environ Heal, vol. 211, nr. 3–4, 2008, pp. 326–336.
6. X. Querol, A. Alastuey,T. Moreno, M.M. Viana, S. Castillo , J. Pey , S. Rodríguez, B. Artiñano, P. Salvador, M. Sánchez, S. Garcia Dos Santos, M.D. Herce Garraleta, R. Fernandez-Patier, S. Moreno-Grau, L. Negral, M.C. Minguillón, E. Monfort, M.J. Sanz, R. Palomo-Marín, E. Pinilla-Gil, E. Cuevas, J. De la Rosa, A. Sanchez de la Campa, "Spatial and temporal variations in airborne particulate matter (PM10 and PM2.5) across Spain 1999– 2005", Atmos Environ, vol. 42, n.17, 2008, pp. 3964–79.
7. T.F. Mar, G.A. Norris, J.Q. Koenig, T.V. Larson, "Associations between air pollution and mortality in Phoenix, 1995-1997". Environ Health Persp., vol. 108, 2000, pp. 347-353.
8. B.D. Ostro, S. Hurley, M.J. Lipsett, "Air pollution and daily mortality in the Coachella Valley, California: a study of PM10 dominated by coarse particles". Environ. Res., vol. 81, 1999, pp. 231-238.
9. A. Alastuey,T. Moreno, M.M. Viana, S. Castillo , J. Pey , S. Rodríguez, B. Artiñano, P. Salvador, M. Sánchez, S. Garcia Dos Santos, M.D. Herce Garraleta, R. Fernandez- Patier, S. Moreno-Grau, L. Negral, M.C. Minguillón, E. Monfort, M.J. Sanz, R. Palomo- Marín, E. Pinilla-Gil et al, " Spatial and temporal variations in airborne particulate matter (PM10 and PM2.5) across Spain 1999– 2005", Atmos Environ, vol. 42, n.17, 2008, pp. 3964–79.
10. L. Perez, A. Tobías, X. Querol, J. Pey, A. Alastuey, J. Díaz, J. Sunyer, "Saharan dust, particulate matter and cause-specific mortality: A case–crossover study in Barcelona (Spain)", Environ. Intern., vol. 48, 2012, pp. 150–155.

11. L. Perez, A. Tobias, X. Querol, N. Künzli, J. Pey, A. Alastuey, M. Viana, N. Valero, M. Gonzales-Cabre, J. Suney "Coarse particles from Saharan dust and daily mortality", Epidemiology, vol. 19, n. 6, 2008, pp. 800–7.
12. Web site source: http://ec.europa.eu/environment/air/quality/standards.htm
13. R. Esworthy, "Air Quality: EPA's 2013 Changes to the Particulate Matter (PM) Standard", Congressional Research Service 7-5700, n. R42934 , 2013, p. 6.
14. B. Srimuruganandam, S. Nagendra, "Source characterization of PM10 and PM2.5 mass using a chemical mass balance model at urban roadside", Sci Total Environ., vol. 433, 2012, pp. 8-19.
15. Ragazzi, M., Rada, E.C., "Multi-step approach for comparing the local air pollution contributions of conventional and innovative MSW thermo-chemical treatments", Chemosphere, vol. 89, nr. 6, 2012, pp. 694-701.
16. S. Ciuta, M. Schiavon, A. Chistè, M. Ragazzi, E.C. Rada, M. Tubino, A. Badea, T. Apostol, "Role of feedstock transport in the balance of primary PM emissions in two case-studies: RMSW incineration vs. sintering plant". Sci. Bull. Mechan Eng., series D, vol. 74, nr. 1, 2012, pp. 211-218.
17. Ionescu G., Zardi D., Tirler W., Rada E.C., Ragazzi M., "A critical analysis of emissions and atmospheric dispersion of pollutants from plants for the treatment of residual municipal solid waste", Sci. Bull. Mechan Eng, Series D, vol. 74, nr. 4, 2012, pp. 227-240.
18. J. Kukkonena, M. Pohjolaa, R.S. Sokhib, L. Luhanab, N. Kitwiroonb, L. Fragkoub, M. Rantamäkia, E. Bergec, V. Ødegaardd, L.H. Slørdale, B. Denbye, S. Finardif , "Analysis and evaluation of selected local-scale PM10 air pollution episodes in four European cities: Helsinki, London, Milan and Oslo", Atmos Environ, vol. 39, n. 15, 2005, pp. 2759–2773.
19. A. Răducanu, E. Codorean, C. Grigoriu, A. Meghea, "Physical chemical characteristics of power plant emissions and their impact on human health", Sci. Bull. Chem Material Sci., series B, vol. 73, nr. 2, 2011, pp. 115-122.
20. X. Querol, A. Alastuey, M.M. Viana,S. Rodriguez, B. Artiñano, P. Salvador, S. Garcia do Santos, R. Fernandez Patier, C.R. Ruiz, J. de la Rosa, A. Sanchez de la Campa, M. Menendez, J.I. Gil, "Speciation and origin of PM10 and PM2.5 in Spain", J Aerosol Sci, vol. 35, n.9, 2004, p.1151–72.
21. X. Querol, A. Alastuey,T. Moreno, M.M. Viana, S. Castillo , J. Pey , S. Rodríguez, B. Artiñano, P. Salvador, M. Sánchez, S. Garcia Dos Santos, M.D. Herce Garraleta, R. Fernandez-Patier, S. Moreno-Grau, L. Negral, M.C. Minguillón, E. Monfort, M.J. Sanz, R. Palomo-Marín, E. Pinilla-Gil et al, " Spatial and temporal variations in airborne particulate matter (PM10 and PM2.5) across Spain 1999– 2005", Atmos Environ., vol. 42, n.17, 2008, pp. 3964–79.
22. C. Misra, M.D. Geller, P. Shah, C. Sioutas, P.A. Solomon, "Development and evaluation of a continuous coarse (PM10-PM2.5) particle monitor". J Air Waste Manage. Assoc., vol. 51, 2001, pp. 1309-1317.
23. K. Cheung, N. Daher, W. Kam, M.M. Shafer, Z. Ning, J.J. Schauer, C. Sioutas, Spatial and temporal variation of chemical composition and mass closure of ambient coarse particulate matter (PM10-2.5) in the Los Angeles area, Atmos Environ., vol. 45, 2011, pp. 2651-2662.

24. M. Sillanpää, R. Hillamo, S. Saarikoski, A. Frey, A. Pennanen, U. Makkonen, Z. Spolnik, R. Van Grieken, M. Branis, B. Brunekreef, M.C. Chalbot, T. Kuhlbusch, J. Sunyer, V.M. Kerminen, M. Kulmala, R.O. Salonen, "Chemical composition and mass closure of particulate matter at six urban sites in Europe", Atmos Environ., vol. 40, 2006, pp. 212–223.
25. C. Hueglin, R. Gehrig, U. Baltensperger, M. Gysel, C. Monn, H. Vonmont, "Chemical characterisation of PM2.5, PM10 and coarse particles at urban, near-city and rural sites in Switzerland", Atmos Environ., vol. 39, 2005, pp. 637–651.
26. D. Hjortenkrans, B. Bergbäck, A. Häggerud, "New metal emission patterns in road traffic environments", Environ Monit Assess, vol. 117, 2006, pp. 85–98.
27. A.P. Davis, M. Shokouhiian, S. Ni, "Loading estimates of lead, copper, cadmium, and zinc in urban runoff from specific sources", Chemosphere, vol. 44, 2001, pp. 997–1009.
28. E.C. Rada, M. Ragazzi, E. Malloci, "Role of levoglucosan as a tracer of wood combustion in an alpine region", Environ Technol., vol. 33, n. 9, 2012, pp. 989–994.
29. J.P. Putaud, F. Raes, R. Van Dingenen, E. Brüggemann, M.C. Facchini, S. Decesari, S. Fuzzi, R. Gehrig, C. Hüglin, P. Laj, G. Lorbeer, W. Maenhaut, N. Mihalopoulos, K. Müller, X. Querol, S. Rodriguez, J. Schneider, G. Spindler, H. ten Brink, K. Tørseth, A. Wiedensohler, "AEuropean aerosol phenomenology-2: chemical characteristics of particulate matter at kerbside, urban, rural and background sites in Europe", Atmos Environ., vol. 38, 2004, pp. 2579–2595.
30. K. Juda-Rezlera, M. Reizera, J.P. Oudinetb, "Determination and analysis of PM10 source apportionment during episodes of air pollution in Central Eastern European urban areas: The case of wintertime 2006", vol. 45, n. 36, 2011, pp. 6557–6566.
31. P. Aarnio, J. Martikainen, T. Hussein, I. Valkama, H. Vehkamäki, L. Sogacheva, J. Härkönen, A. Karppinen, T. Koskentalo, J. Kukkonen, M. Kulmala, "Analysis and evaluation of selected PM10 pollution episodes in the Helsinki Metropolitan Area in 2002", Atmos Environ., vol. 42, n. 17, 2008, pp. 3992-4005.
32. M. Koçaka, N. Mihalopoulosb, N. Kubilaya, "Contributions of natural sources to high PM10 and PM2.5 events in the eastern Mediterranean", Atmos Environ., vol. 41, n. 18, 2007, pp. 3806–3818.
33. E. Fridella, M. Ferma, A. Ekbergb, "Emissions of particulate matters from railways – Emission factors and condition monitoring", Transport Res. Part D: Trans. Env, vol. 15, 2010, pp. 240–245.
34. M. Ragazzi, M, Grigoriu, E.C. Rada, E. Malloci, F. Natolino, "Health risk assessment from combustion of sewage sludge treatment: three caste study comparison", Proceedings of the Internationl Conference on Risk Management, Assessment and Mitigation- RIMA'10, 2010, pp.176-180
35. E.C. Rada, I. A. Istrate, M. Ragazzi, "Trends in the management of the Residual Municipal Solid Waste", Environ Technol., vol. 30, nr. 7, 2009, pp. 651-661.
36. M. Ragazzi, E.C. Rada, "Effect of recent strategies of selective collection on the design of municipal solid waste treatment plants in Italy", WIT Transactions on Ecology and the environment, vol. 109, 2008, pp. 613-620.
37. M. Ragazzi, E.C. Rada, "RDF/SRF evolution and MSW bio-drying", WIT Transactions on Ecology and Environment, vol. 163, 2012, pp. 199-208.

38. E.C. Rada, M. Ragazzi, T. Apostol, "Role of Refuse Derived Fuel in the Romanian industrial sector after the entrance in EU", WIT Transactions on Ecology and Environment, vol. 109, 2008, pp. 89-96.
39. E.C. Rada, M. Ragazzi, V. Panaitescu, T. Apostol, "Some research perspectives on emissions from bio-mechanical treatments of municipal solid waste in Europe", Environ Technol., vol. 26, n. 11, 2005, pp. 1297-1302.
40. C. di Mauro, S. Buochon, V. Torretta, "Industrial risk in the lombardy region (Italy): What people perceive and what are the gaps to improve the risk communication and the participatory processes", Chem Eng Transaction, vol. 26, pp. 297-302.
41. F. Amato, X. Querol, A. Alastuey, M. Pandolfi, T. Moreno, J. Gracia, Rodriguez, "Evaluating urban PM10 pollution benefit induced by street cleaning activities", Atmos Environ., vol. 43, n. 29, 2009, pp. 4472–4480.
42. C.M. Chou, Y.M. Chang, W.Y. Lin, C.H. Tseng, L. Chen, "Evaluation of street sweeping and washing to reduce ambient PM10", Int J Environ Pollut., vol. 31, n. 3–4, 2007, pp. 431–438.
43. R. Langston, R.S.J. Merle, D. Hart, V. Etyemezian, H. Kuhns, H. Gillies, D. Fitz, K. Bumiller, D.E. James, "The preferred alternative method for measuring paved road dust emissions for emissions inventories: mobile technologies vs. The traditional ap-42 methodology". Prepared for EPA OAQPS, March, 2008, pp. 110.
44. H. Taha, "The potential for air-temperature impact from large-scale deployment of solar photovoltaic arrays in urban area", Solar Energy, 2012, http://dx.doi.org/10.1016/j.solener.2012.09.014.
45. C.L Myun, K. Choi, J. Kim, Y. Lim, J Lee, S. Park, "Comparative study of regulated and unregulated toxic emissions characteristics from a spark ignition direct injection light-duty vehicle fueled with gasoline and liquid phase LPG (liquefied petroleum gas)", Energy, vol. 44, 2012, pp. 189 - 196.
46. E.C. Rada, M. Ragazzi, M. Brini, L. Marmo, P. Zambelli, M. Chelodi, M. Ciolli, "Perspectives of low-cost sensors adoption for air quality monitoring". Sci Bull. Mechan Eng. vol. 74, serie D, n. 2, 2012, pp. 243-250.
47. E.C. Rada, M. Grigoriu, M. Ragazzi, P. Fedrizzi, "Web oriented technologies and equipments for MSW collection", Proceedings of the International Conference on Risk Management, Assessment and Mitigation - RIMA '10, 201, pp. 150-153
48. V. Torretta V., E.C. Rada, V.N. Panaitescu, T. Apostol "Some considerations on particulate generated by traffic, Sci Bull. Mechan Eng., vol. 74, serie D, n. 4, 2012, pp. 141-148.

CHAPTER 3

Application of Strategies for Particulate Matter Reduction in Urban Areas: An Italian Case

VINCENZO TORRETTA, MASSIMO RABONI, SABRINA COPELLI, ELENA CRISTINA RADA, MARCO RAGAZZI, GABRIELA IONESCU, TIBERIU APOSTOL, AND ADRIAN BADEA

3.1 INTRODUCTION

In the past 15 years the concentrations of particulate matter (PM) in Europe is decreasing [1], although they are still very common situations exceeding the thresholds set by the new regulations. Northern Italy is one of the most polluted in Europe. Italian PM10 emissions begin to decline from 1994 and from that year showed a 30% decrease. The road transport sector in the last three years has contributed to the total emissions as the second emissive share (about 20%), while industrial combustion represents the 35% of total emissions. Compared with the data obtained in 2008 emissions of PM10 decreased of the 11%. The most significant contributions to the reduction of emissions of this pollutant are related to the non-industrial combustion (-12%), road transport (-7%) and combustion in industry (-25%). The reduction in the field of civil heating is due not only to the reduction in the consumption of wood, but also to the change of the emission factors [2,3,4].

Studies carried out by the WHO [4] demonstrate the negative effects of particulate matter on cardiovascular and respiratory systems (e.g. lung cancer), as well as premature deaths, acute and chronic diseases, decrease in life expectancy and reproduction capacity. The European Environment Agency [1] has estimated that each year in Europe smog kills about 310,000 people, of whom 50,000 in Italy alone; geographical areas most exposed to pollution are the Po Valley (where deaths from smog are around 7,000 per year) and the European macro-region consists of Belgium, the Netherlands and Luxembourg. The WHO [4] stated that the reduction in atmospheric levels of PM10 annual average of 70 to 20 $\mu g/m^3$ (or PM2.5 from 35 to 10 $\mu g/m^3$) would decrease by 15% the number of deaths due to air pollution.

The causes of air pollution in urban areas are mainly vehicular traffic and heating of buildings, areas in which action is required through concrete solutions for production facilities and power plants, energy efficiency policies of the buildings, diffusion of renewable and clean sources for energy production and for heating homes and a new mobility focused on local public transport and railways [5].

According to the ranking of Legambiente, in 2011, there were as many as 55 Italian cities that exceeded the daily limits introduced by Italian Law 155/2010 as regards the levels of particulate air pollution. In the light of the revision of the European legislation [6,7], the situation will get worse.

The paper presents the case study of Varese, a city in the Northern part of Lombardy (Italy), which in 2012 has gone beyond the PM10 tolerance threshold for 44 times. After the analysis of the geographic and meteorological conditions of the city, the time series of PM concentration has been evaluated in order to locate spatial and temporal critical situation. Therefore, emissions inventory from different sources has been created in order to find the major sources. Finally, some strategies in order to reduce critical situation have been proposed and assessed from the environmental and economic point of view.

3.2 MATERIAL AND METHODS

3.2.1 CASE STUDY

Varese has about 79,000 inhabitants and a population density of 1,500 inhab/km^2. The settlements stands between about 240 and 460 m a.s.l. in different valleys and downtown is at about 382 m a.s.l.. The weather is rainy and is characterized by a prevailing wind with N-S direction and (Fig. 1). Average daily temperature are below 10°C for about 160 d/y (Fig. 2).

Nevertheless, the city has serious problems of particulate matter pollution, in particular in the downtown zone. Indeed in Fig. 3 the dynamics of PM10 from 2008 to 2012 are reported showing significant peaks in winter.

Meteorological data coming from different stations have been used to evaluate atmospheric stability, useful to understand possible critical situation for air pollution.

3.2.2 EMISSIONS ASSESSMENT

Emissions have been firstly evaluated by the means of INEMAR inventory of emissions [9]. INEMAR gives aggregated data regarding the whole municipality. Therefore, a further investigation regarding, in particular, non-industrial heating, road and train transport has been carried out in order to locate sourced in the 19 zones of the city (Fig. 4).

3.2.3 THEORETICAL APPROACH

Emission factors for road traffic from EME/CORINAIR emission inventory [11,12] have been used and coupled with COPERT software [13]. Road traffic behavior has been extracted from field investigation in several roads inside the city [10] and considering the current procedure for management (sweeping, washing, etc) [14,15,16,17,18]. The car fleet has been taken into account considering the available data [19].

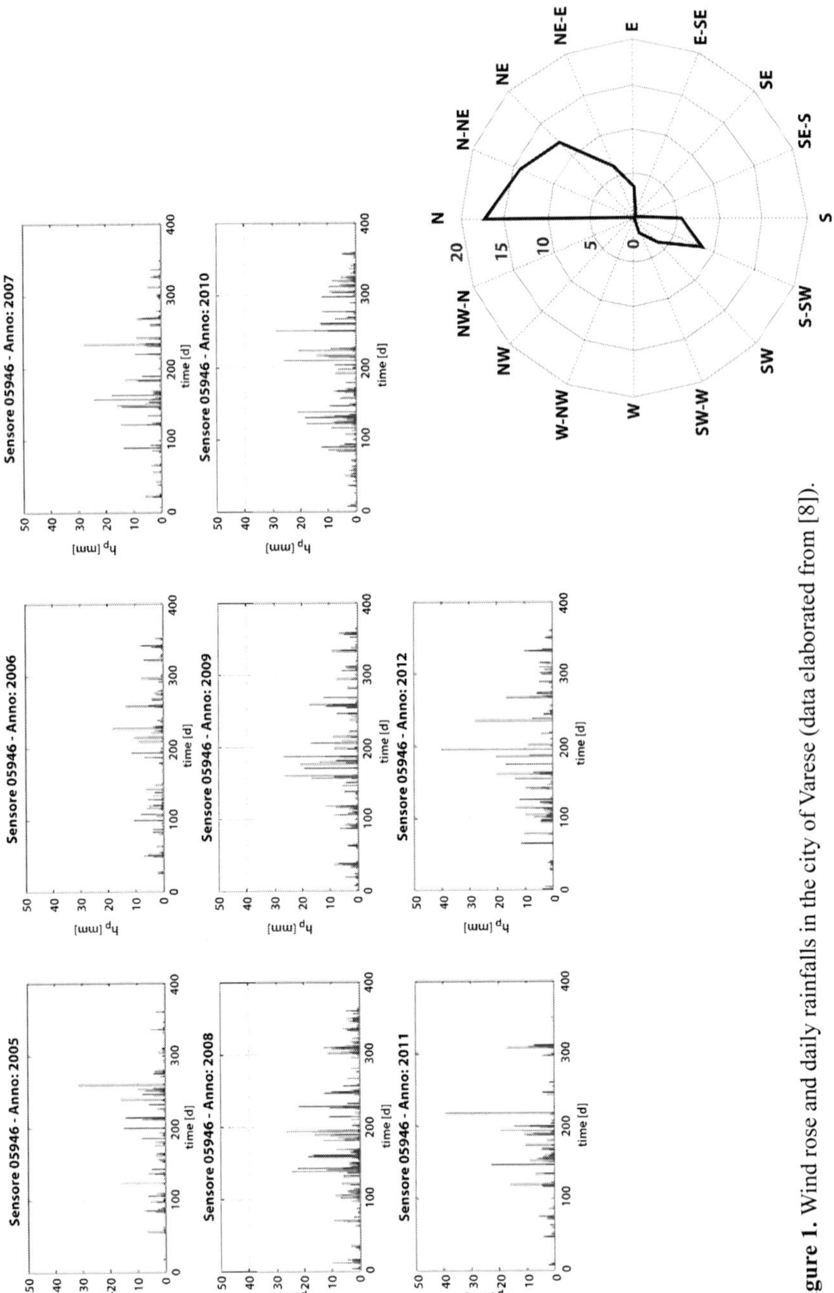

Figure 1. Wind rose and daily rainfalls in the city of Varese (data elaborated from [8]).

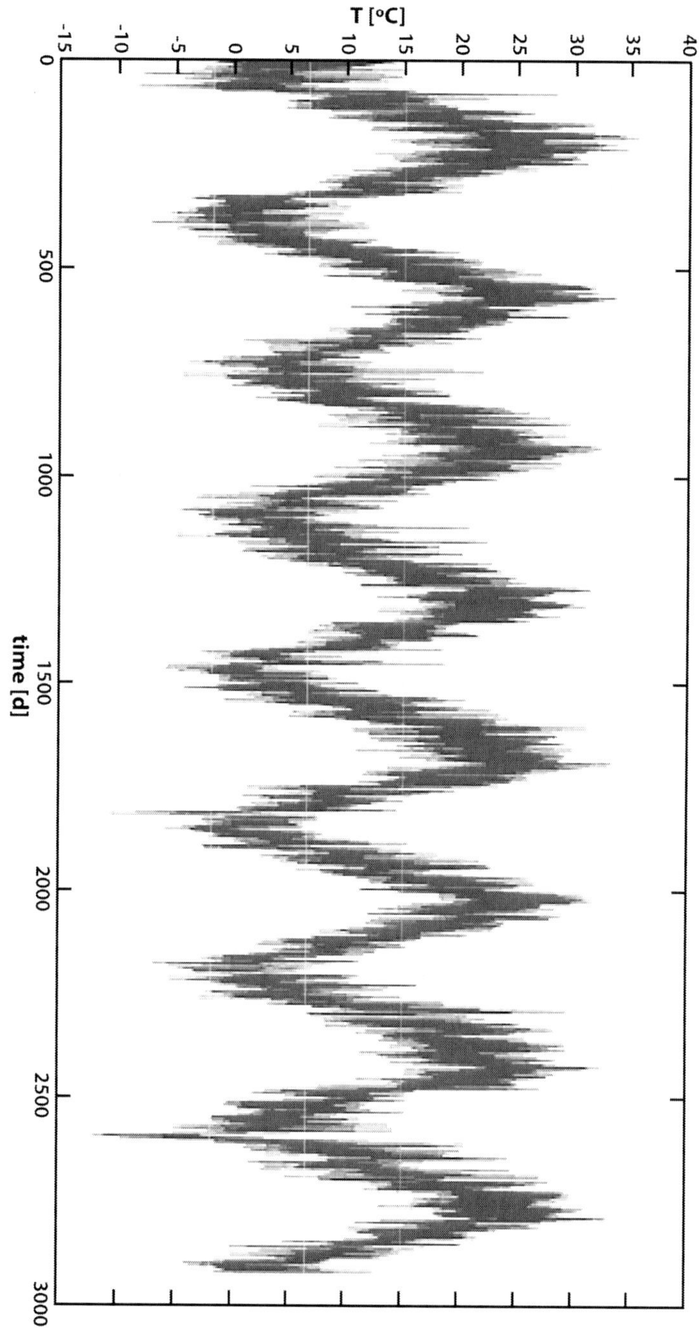

Figure 2. Hourly average temperature in the city of Varese (data elaborated from [8]).

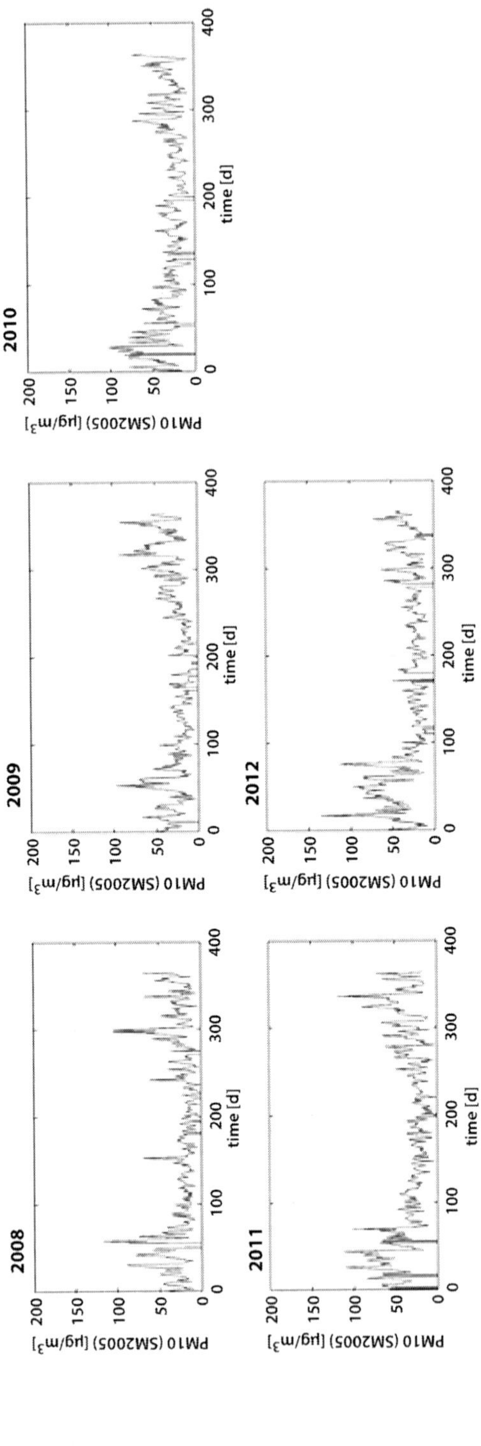

Figure. 3. PM10 concentration in Varese downtown (data elaborated from [8]).

About non-industrial heating, investigation on local authorities allowed to distribute the boilers type, fuel into the cities (CENED) [8].

3.3 RESULTS AND DISCUSSION

In Varese, global emissions of particulate matter are caused by non- industrial combustion (about 74%; above all, heating) and road transport (about 24%) [8]. In general we can consider as negligible all the contributions different from heating systems and traffic (Fig. 5). Anyway, it would be necessary underline that the theoretical approach in case of industrial emissions, needs to be focused considering some important aspect regard-

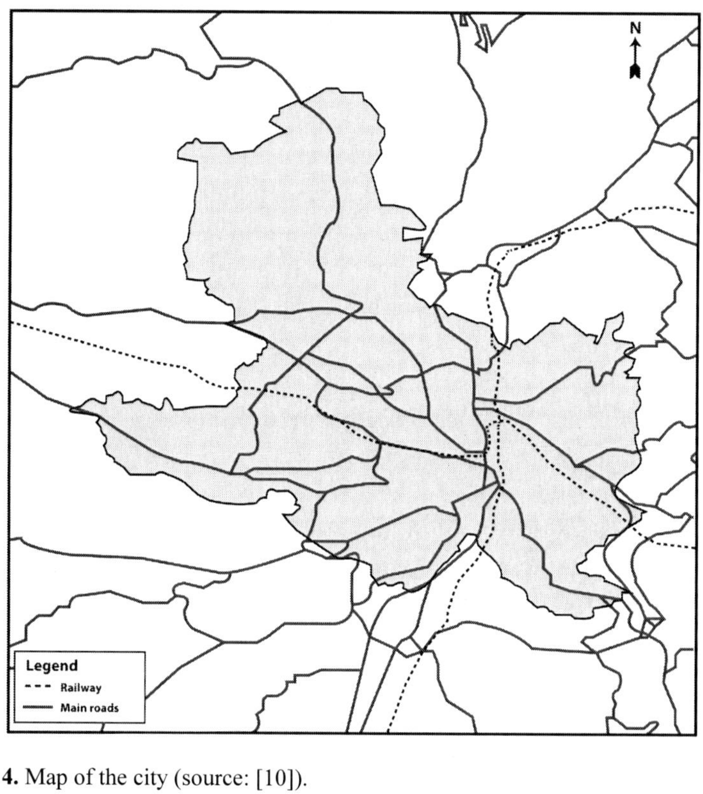

Figure 4. Map of the city (source: [10]).

ing the modality of emission in atmosphere of the exhaust treated airs. For instance, considering the biofiltration processes for treatment of exhaust air characterized by presence of dust and VOCs, it could be important the difference between the areal contribution of a classical biofilter compared with the piped effluent from a biotrickling filter with a punctual emission [20,21]. Also the stack height of a punctual emission can play an important role in decreasing the human exposure to air pollutants [22,23]. However the exposure pathways must be considered with particular attention as persistent pollutants can emerge in matrices different from the one of the original release (atmosphere) [24,25,26]. Recent approaches try to integrate the conventional monitoring strategy in order to make more clear the real impact of the emissions of modern plants [27].

In order to solve the problem, the main issue has to be faced: non-industrial combustion. It is necessary, therefore, to put adequate attention to the heating and new technologies that we have to reduce these emission values, given that 64% of Varese households have obsolete boilers, which cause a waste of heat energy equal to about 10Mtep annual per system [8]. The modernization of these plants fueled by a cost to the public, would save each year to EUR 16.3 billion and avoid the unnecessary emission. It is calculated that by replacing old boilers with modern condensing systems in 10% of apartment buildings, the city would have an environmental impact equivalent to -30% in terms of PM emissions. It is to perform actions such as increasing the insulation in the walls and to replace the windows, put the blinds on the windows, use of heat pumps and solar energy [11].

Additionally, the sector of domestic wood combustion needs a particular attention as old stoves can give a contribution of PM10 that can be dominant in specific areas [28].

Road traffic and related emissions can be reduced by new rules in urban mobility and road conditions, reducing the 10% of the PM. Also rules connected with change of atmospheric stability can be a solutions, but they require a parking and a public transport system able to manage such situations.

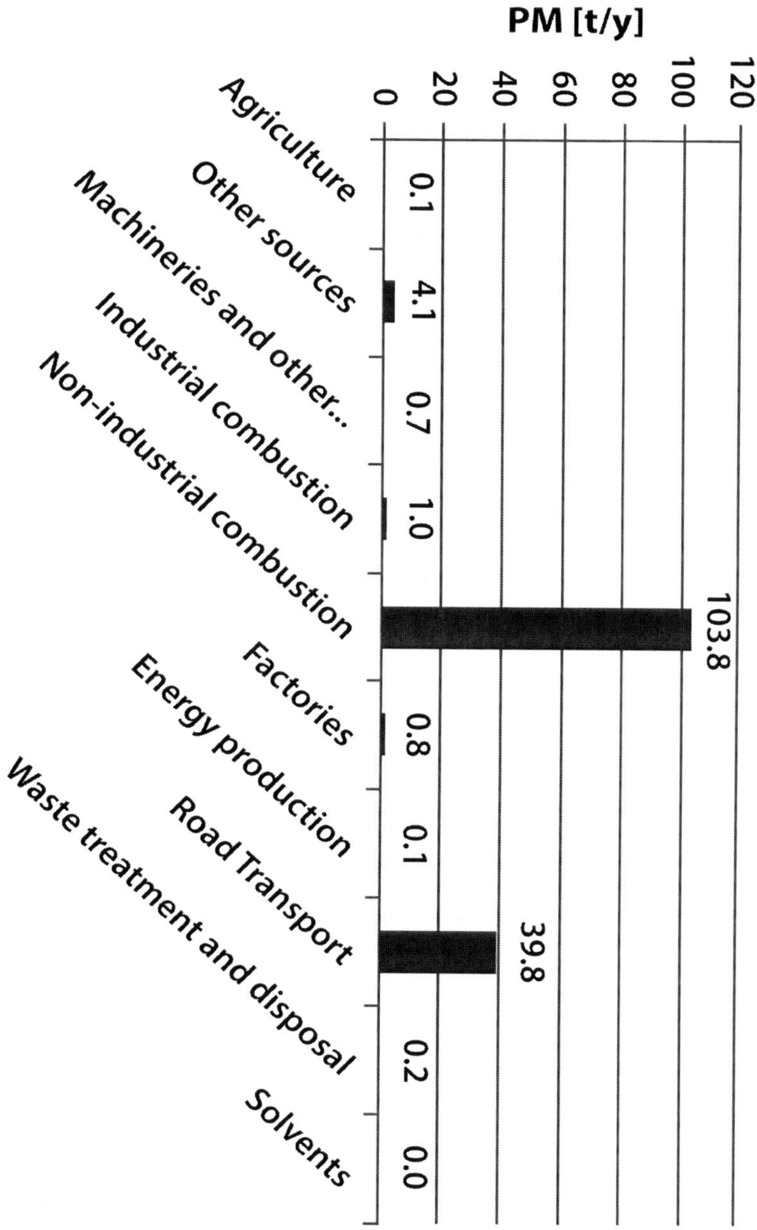

Figure 5. Emission sources in the city of Varese.

3.4 CONCLUSIONS

The paper presents the case of particulate matter pollution of Varese, a Northern-Italian city. The cause of this pollution is connected manly to non-industrial combustion due to house heating and, for one fourth, by road transport.

Possible solutions with their environmental and economic impact have been presented, also considering weather conditions.

We must therefore pay close attention to local politics that should not only think about emergency response to reach a legal limit, an end in itself, but rather a long-term policy that aims to reduce smog and protect the health of citizens thus improving the quality of life.

REFERENCES

1. EEA – European Environment Agency, "Air quality in Europe – 2012 report", Copenhagen, 2012.
2. G. Ionescu, T. Apostol, E.C. Rada, M. Ragazzi, V. Torretta, "Critical analysis of strategies for PM reduction in urban areas", Sci. Bull., series D, vol. 75, nr. 2, 2013, pp. 175-186.
3. G. Tsilingiridis, T. Zachariadis, Z. Samaras, "Spatial and temporal characteristics of air pollutant emissions in Thessaloniki, Greece: investigation of emission abatement measures", Sci. Total Environ., vol. 300, n. 1-3, pp. 99-113, 2002.
4. World Health Organization (WHO) Europe, "Air Quality Guidelines – Global Update 2005 – Particulate matter, ozone, nitrogen dioxide and sulfur dioxide", Copenhagen, 2006, ISBN 92 890 2192 6.
5. E. Fridella, M. Ferma, A. Ekbergb, "Emissions of particulate matters from railways – Emission factors and condition monitoring", Transport Res. Part D: Trans. Environ., vol. 15, 2010, pp. 240–245.
6. J.P. Putaud, F. Raes, R. Van Dingenen, E. Brüggemann, M.C. Facchini, S. Decesari, S. Fuzzi, R. Gehrig, C. Hüglin, P. Laj, G. Lorbeer, W. Maenhaut, N. Mihalopoulos, K. Müller, X. Querol, S. Rodriguez, J. Schneider, G. Spindler, H. ten Brink, K. Tørseth, A. Wiedensohler, "A European aerosol phenomenology-2: chemical characteristics of particulate matter at kerbside, urban, rural and background sites in Europe", Atmos Environ., vol. 38, 2004, pp. 2579–2595.
7. R. Esworthy, "Air Quality: EPA's 2013 Changes to the Particulate Matter (PM) Standard", Congressional Research Service 7-5700, n. R42934 , 2013, p. 6.
8. Agenzia Regionale Per l'Ambiente (ARPA) Lombardia, http://ita.arpalombardia.it/ita/index.asp. Last access: June 2013.

9. INEMAR- INventario EMissioni Aria, Agenzia Regionale per la Protezione dell'Ambiente, http://www.arpalombardia.it/inemar/inemarhome.htm, Last access: May, 2013
10. Municipality of Varese (Italy), "Urban mobility plan – General Report (Draft)", 2011.
11. V. Torretta, E.C. Rada, V. Panaitescu, T. Apostol, "Some considerations on particulate generated by traffic", Sci. Bull. Mechan Eng., series D, vol. 74, nr. 4, 2012, pp. 241-248.
12. EEA - European Environmental Agency, EMEP/CORINAIR Emission Inventory Guidebook. Technical report No 9, 2009, revision March 2013.
13. Emisia, COPERT 4 v.10.0 Manual, http://www.emisia.com/copert/, 2012.
14. F. Amato, X. Querol , C. Johansson, C. Nagl, A. Alastuey, "A review on the effectiveness ofstreet sweeping, washing and dust suppressants as urban PM control methods". Sci. Total Environ., vol. 408, 2010, pp. 3070–3084.
15. F. Amato, X. Querol, A. Alastuey, M. Pandolfi, T. Moreno, J. Gracia, Rodriguez, "Evaluating urban PM10 pollution benefit induced by street cleaning activities", Atmos Environ., vol. 43, n. 29, 2009, pp. 4472–4480.
16. C.M. Chou, Y.M. Chang, W.Y. Lin, C.H. Tseng, L. Chen, "Evaluation of street sweeping and washing to reduce ambient PM10", Int J Environ Pollut., vol. 31, n. 3–4, 2007, pp. 431–438.
17. R. Langston, R.S.J. Merle, D. Hart, V. Etyemezian, H. Kuhns, H. Gillies, D. Fitz, K. Bumiller,D.E. James, "The preferred alternative method for measuring paved road dust emissions for emissions inventories: mobile technologies vs. The traditional ap-42 methodology". Prepared for EPA OAQPS, March, 2008, pp. 110.
18. C.A. Alexandrescu, M.C. Surugiu, "Experimental study on the influence of traffic on pollutants in a street canyon from Bucharest", Sci. Bull., D, vol. 73, n.1, 2011, pp. 191-204.
19. ACI, http://www.aci.it/sezione-istituzionale/studi-e-ricerche/dati-e-statistiche/autoritratto-2012.html, Last access: May 2013
20. S. Copelli, V. Torretta, M. Raboni, P. Viotti, A. Luciano, G. Mancini, G. Nano G., "Improving biotreatment efficiency of hot waste air streams: experimental upgrade of a fullplant", Chem Eng Trans., vol. 30, 2012, pp. 49-54.
21. V. Torretta, M. Raboni, S. Copelli, P. Caruson, "Application of multi-stage biofilter pilot plants to remove odor and VOCs from industrial activities air emissions", Proceedings of Energy and Sustainability 2013, 19 – 21 June, Bucharest, Romania.
22. M. Ragazzi, W. Tirler, G. Angelucci, D. Zardi, E.C. Rada, "Management of atmospheric pollutants from waste incineration processes: The case of Bozen", Waste Manage Research, vol. 31, n. 3, 2013, pp. 235-240.
23. M. Ragazzi, E.C. Rada, "Multi-step approach for comparing the local air pollution contributions of conventional and innovative MSW thermo-chemical treatments", Chemosphere, vol. 89, n. 6, 2012, pp. 694-701.
24. V. Torretta, A. Katsoyiannis, "Occurrence of polycyclic aromatic hydrocarbons in sludges from different stages of a wastewater treatment plant in Italy", Environ Technol., vol. 34, n. 7, 2013, pp. 937-943.

25. V. Torretta, "PAHs in wastewater: Removal efficiency in a conventional wastewater treatment plant and comparison with model predictions", Environ. Technol., vol. 33, n. 8, 2012, pp. 851-855.
26. A. Luciano, P. Viotti, V. Torretta, G. Mancini, "Numerical approach to modelling pulse- mode soil flushing on a Pb-contaminated soil", J. Soils Sediments, vol. 13, n. 1, 2013, pp. 43-55.
27. E.C. Rada, M. Ragazzi, M. Brini, L. Marmo, P. Zambelli, M. Chelodi, M. Ciolli, "Perspectives of low-cost sensors adoption for air quality monitoring", Sci Bull., series D, vol. 74, 2012, pp. 243-250.
28. E.C. Rada, M. Ragazzi, E. Malloci "Role of levoglucosan as a tracer of wood combustion in an alpine region", Environ Technol., vol. 33, n. 9, 2012, pp. 989-994.

CHAPTER 4

Infrastructure and Automobile Shifts: Positioning Transit to Reduce Life-Cycle Environmental Impacts for Urban Sustainability Goals

MIKHAIL CHESTER, STEPHANIE PINCETL, ZOE ELIZABETH, WILLIAM EISENSTEIN, AND JUAN MATUTE

4.1 BACKGROUND

It is widely accepted that the combustion from passenger vehicle tailpipes is a leading cause of environmental pollution and emerging life-cycle approaches present an opportunity to better understand how transit investments reduce transportation impacts. In California, automobile travel is responsible for 38% of statewide greenhouse gas (GHG) emissions and other pollutants have been linked to significant health impacts [1, 2]. California's Assembly Bill 32 calls for the reduction of statewide GHG emissions to 1990 levels by 2020. To achieve this, a suite of strategies will be deployed, including Senate Bill 375 which requires regional transportation plans to achieve GHG emissions targets from the transportation system and may induce cities to deploy new public transit systems.

Passenger vehicles, however, do not exist in isolation as they require a large and complex system to support a vehicle's operation. To understand the environmental impacts from transportation systems, and more importantly how to cost-effectively minimize these impacts, it is necessary to include vehicle, infrastructure, and energy production life-cycle components, in addition to operation [3]. A life-cycle approach is particularly important for new mass transit systems that produce large upfront impacts during the deployment of new infrastructure systems for long-run benefits in the reduction of automobile travel [4]. However, little is known about the life-cycle environmental benefits and costs of deploying public transit systems to meet urban energy and environmental goals. Using the city of Los Angeles as a case study, a life-cycle assessment (LCA) of the Orange bus rapid transit (BRT) and Gold light rail transit (LRT) lines is developed. These transit lines, both deployed in the past decade, provide an opportunity to better understand how new transit systems will help cities reduce transportation impacts.

4.2 METHODOLOGY

An environmental LCA is developed for the Orange BRT, Gold LRT, and competing automobile trips. The LCA includes vehicle (e.g., manufacturing and maintenance), infrastructure (e.g., construction and operation), and energy production components, in addition to vehicle propulsion effects [3]. To inform a broad array of transportation policy and decision makers, two different LCA framings are used: attributional and consequential. The attributional framing evaluates the long-run average footprint of each system allocating impacts to a passenger-mile-traveled (PMT). It includes, for example, the construction impacts of the existing road system for an automobile trip. However, given the importance of understanding how public transit investments contribute to urban sustainability goals, a consequential analysis of the decision to build each system is also produced, culminating in a cumulative impact savings at some future time. The consequential analysis answers how the BRT and LRT systems may contribute to Los Angeles (LA) meeting its Senate Bill 375 GHG and air quality goals. The results from the attributional and consequential approaches should be considered independently.

4.2.1 LIFE-CYCLE CHARACTERISTICS OF LOS ANGELES TRANSPORTATION SYSTEMS

The LCA methods used follow those reported in existing research by the authors, however, significant efforts were made to obtain system-specific data from LA Metro [5] and model life-cycle impacts with regionalized energy mixes and processes. Extensive details are provided in Chester et al [6] and the following discussion focuses on the data collection and methods used to assess the dominating life-cycle processes. For each mode, near-term (at maturity, in the 2020–2030 time period) and long-term (2030–2050) vehicles are modeled.

4.2.1.1 ORANGE LINE BRT

The Orange BRT is an 18 mile dedicated right-of-way running east–west through the San Fernando Valley. The line opened in 2005 and now services 25 500 riders per day, exceeding initial forecasts [7]. The line is viewed as a tremendous success; service has been increased to meet the latent demand, its construction has induced 140 000 new annual bike trips on the buffering green belt, and has roused development [8–10]. The initial line consists of a two-lane asphalt roadway connecting 18 stations, sometimes buffered by landscaping. In 2012 a 4 mile extension from Canoga Park to Chatsworth was opened. Orange BRT buses are 60 foot compressed natural gas (CNG) articulated North American Bus Industry vehicles with the structure, chassis, and suspension (54% of weight) manufactured in Hungary and final assembly occurring in Alabama [5]. Vehicle manufacturing is assessed with Ecoinvent's bus manufacturing processes using current and projected European mixes [11–13]. The buses use conventional lead-acid batteries with an expected lifetime of 13 months [5]. The energy and emissions effects from ocean going vessel transport (Hungary to Alabama) and driving the buses from Alabama to LA are included [14]. LA Metro expects buses to last 15 years [5]. Engineering design documents are used to determine busway characteristics. The western-most segment of the line uses local roadways and the 17 mile dedicated busway consists of roughly 13 miles of asphalt and 4 miles of concrete surface layers. Recycled materials were used for the subbase. Asphalt wearing layers, concrete wearing layers, and the subbase are modeled with PaLATE [15] and are assumed to have 20, 15, and 100 year lifetimes. Stations are also included and are designed as a raised concrete platform [16]. The construction and maintenance of the 4700 parking spaces are also assessed with PaLATE. The Orange BRT line uses 1.2 GWh of electricity [5] purchased from LA Department of Water and Power (LADWP) for infrastructure operation including roadway, station, and parking lot lighting, and is evaluated with GREET [14]. Routine maintenance of vehicles and infrastructure are modeled with SimaPro [13].

Orange BRT vehicle operation effects are based on emissions testing by the California Air Resources Board (CARB) of similar bus engines [17, 18]. CARB results for urban duty drive cycles are used and assume that buses will use three way catalysts in the near-term. The emission profiles are validated against other testing reports for similar vehicles and engines [19–28]. In the long-term, it is assumed that Orange BRT buses will achieve fuel economies consistent with best available technology buses today (effectively a 23% improvement from today's buses) and that the CARB 2020 certification standards are met which require 75–85% reductions in air pollutants [17]. The extraction, processing, transport, and distribution of CNG for the buses are evaluated with GREET [14] including upstream effects.

4.2.1.2 GOLD LINE LRT

The Gold line is an expanding rail system that extends from downtown LA to east LA and Pasadena, with plans to triple the line length in the coming decades. The system began operation in 2003 and currently consists of

19.7 mile of at-grade, retained fill, open cut, and aerial sections. LA Metro uses 54 tonne AnsaldoBreda P2550 2-car 76-seat trains manufactured in Italy and shipped by ocean going vessel to LA. Train manufacturing was assessed with SimaPro [13] with current and future European electricity mixes [12] and transport with GREET [14]. The infrastructure assessment is based on engineering design documents [29] which are used to develop a material and construction equipment assessment following the methods used by Chester and Horvath (2009) [4]. The unique construction activities associated with track sections are assessed and detailed characteristics are reported in Chester et al (2012) [6]. There are currently 21 stations of which 19 are at-grade. Satellite imagery is used to determine the area of station platforms which are designed as steel-reinforced concrete slabs on a subbase. The Gold line has 2300 parking spaces across 9 stations, and these are assessed with PaLATE [15]. Electricity consumption data were provided to the research team by LA Metro and are from meters at stations and maintenance yards [5]. In 2010, 20 GWh were purchased from LADWP, 3.2 GWh from Pasadena Water and Power, and 1.2 GWh from Southern California Edison, and propulsion electricity use accounts for roughly one-half of the total [30]. Given the dominating share of LADWP electricity consumed, the utility is used to assess the air emissions of electricity production [14]. Currently, 39% of LADWP electricity is produced from coal and there are plans to phase this fuel out by 2030 as the utility transitions their portfolio towards renewable targets [31]. The 2030 LADWP mix will use more natural gas and renewables and would decrease electricity generation GHG emissions by 50% and SOx by 60% [14]. Vehicle and infrastructure maintenance and insurance impacts are also modeled [6].

Gold line trains consume approximately 10 kWh of electricity per vehicle mile traveled (VMT) [30] and current and future electricity mixes are assessed to determine near-term and long-term vehicle footprints. The 2030 LADWP mix is used for long-term train operation where the generation of propulsion electricity produces fewer GHG and CAP emissions. Primary fuel extraction, processing, and transport to the generation facility (i.e., energy production) effects are modeled with GREET [14].

4.2.1.3 ORANGE BRT AND GOLD LRT INDIRECT AUTOMOBILE EFFECTS

The Orange BRT and Gold LRT lines produce indirect automobile effects through new station access and egress by auto travel. Additionally, the Orange BRT's new biking and walking infrastructure avoids auto trips. The cumulative effect is included in the LCA. 7% of transit riders drive alone to the station and 3% from the stations [9]. These trips are between 1.7 and 2.5 miles [32]. LA Metro [8] estimates that the Orange BRT's biking and walking shift reduces auto annual VMT between 71 000 and 540 000. The indirect auto effects of transit implementation are included in the life-cycle footprint of the Orange BRT and Gold LRT lines, averaged over all PMT.

4.2.1.4 COMPETING AUTOMOBILE TRIP

While LA has an extensive and well-utilized public transportation network, the large sprawling region is dominated by automobile travel at 85% of trips (or 97% of PMT), biking and walking at 13%, and transit at 2% [32]. New transit lines have experienced success in reducing automobile travelers, with (in 2009) 25% of Orange BRT passengers having previously made the trip by auto and 67% of Gold line travelers [9, 33]. Consequently, the assessment of the Orange BRT and Gold LRT lines should consider the life-cycle effects of competing automobile trips to assess the traveler's environmental footprint had transit not existed. The avoided automobile effects are also necessary for evaluating the net change of air pollutants in the region as a result of new transit options.

An automobile trip that substitutes an Orange BRT or Gold LRT line trip is assessed. The transit lines are expected to operate indefinitely so representative automobiles are selected to assess near- (35 mile gallon^{-1}, 3 000 lb) and long-term (54 mile gallon^{-1}, 1800 lb) car travel [14]. The long-term automobile is modeled with a lighter weight to assess technology changes that may be implemented to meet aggressive fuel economy standards. Both automobiles are estimated to have a 160 000 mile lifetime. A transport distance of 2 000 mile from the manufacturing plant to LA is included by class 8b truck. Infrastructure construction is based on a typical LA arterial segment allocated by annual VMT facilitated [34], and modeled with PaLATE [15]. Vehicle insurance and infrastructure construction and maintenance are also included [6].

The near and long-term automobiles are modeled with 35 and 54 mile gallon^{-1} standards in GREET [14] to assess emerging fuel economy standards in the long life expectancy of the new transit systems. Petroleum extraction, processing, and transport effects assuming California Reformulated Gasoline and 16% oil sands are modeled.

4.2.1.5 RIDERSHIP AND MODE SHIFTS

Orange BRT and Gold LRT ridership have been steadily increasing since the lines opened and forecasts for future ridership are developed to assess long-term effects. From its first year of operation to 2009, the Orange BRT has increased yearly boardings from 6.1 to 8.4 million, and the Gold line from 4.8 to 7.6 million [7]. This corresponds to 49 and 55 million PMT in 2009 for the respective systems, an increase of 30% (in 5 years) and 36% (in 7 years). Future ridership estimates are developed using 2035 station access forecasts developed by LA Metro. A polynomial interpolation is used to assess adoption between now and 2035 when an estimated 100 and 130 million annual PMT are delivered by the respective systems [5]. In 2009 the Orange BRT average occupancy was 37 with 57 seats and the Gold line 43 with 72 seats per car [7]. The average occupancy of automobile travel in LA is 1.7 passengers for all trips, 1.4 for households that also use transit, and 1.1 for work trips [32]. Auto trip purpose characteristics are joined with transit onboard survey results and future forecasts to determine avoided automobile travel. Currently, 25% of Orange BRT and 67% of Gold LRT previous trip takers would have made the trip by automobile [9, 33]. Given that fuel prices are expected to increase and the transit lines are expanding to auto dominated regions, may be interconnected with other transit lines [35], and are anticipated to experience further development [10], auto shift forecasts are developed to 2050. Using future trip and station access forecasts from LA Metro, the current auto shift growth rates are extrapolated resulting in a median long-term shift of 52% for the

Orange BRT and 80% for the Gold LRT. Furthermore, to assess avoided automobile travel distance from transit shifts, a clustering approach was used to determine that across household income, workers, and vehicles, one PMT shifted to the Orange BRT or Gold LRT lines avoids one PMT of automobile travel [32, 36].

4.2.2 *ENERGY AND ENVIRONMENTAL INDICATORS AND STRESSORS*

An energy and environmental life-cycle inventory is developed and then joined with photochemical smog formation and human health respiratory impact stressors. The inventory includes end-use energy and emissions of greenhouse gases (GHGs), NO_x, SO_x, CO, PM_{10}, $PM_{2.5}$, and VOCs. GHGs are reported as CO_2-equivalence (CO_{2e}) for a 100 year horizon using radiative forcing multipliers of 25 for CH_4 and 298 for N_2O. Los Angeles has struggled to meet National Ambient Air Quality Standards for PM and ozone so inventory results are joined with impact characterization factors from the Tool for the Reduction and Assessment of Chemical and Other Environmental Impacts (TRACI, v2) to assess respiratory and smog stressors [37]. A stressor is the upper limit of impacts that could occur and not the actual impact that will occur. The deployment of these new transit systems may help LA reduce GHG emissions to meet environmental goals. However, by assessing a broad suite of environmental indicators, unintended tradeoffs (i.e., reducing one impact but increasing another) can be identified early and mitigation strategies developed.

4.3 MODAL PASSENGER MILE COMPARISONS

The Orange BRT and Gold LRT lines will reduce life-cycle per PMT energy use, GHG emissions, and the potential for smog formation at the anticipated near-term and long-term ridership levels. However, given the $PM_{2.5}$ intensity of coal-fired electricity generation powering the Gold LRT, there is a potential for increasing out-of-basin respiratory impacts in the near-term, highlighting the unintended tradeoffs that may occur with disconnected GHG and air quality policies. The Gold LRT respiratory impact potential is the result of coal electricity generation in LADWP's mix and associated mining activities. The coal-fired Navajo Generating Station (NGS) in Arizona and the Intermountain Power Plant (IPP) in Utah are owned, at least in part, by LADWP and the utility is planning to divest in the plants by 2025 [31]. The NGS and IPP are two of the largest coal-fired power plants in the Western US and have been targeted for emissions reductions, primarily to improve visibility at nearby parks including the Grand Canyon [38, 39]. However, secondary particle formation from NO_x and SO_x, in addition to $PM_{2.5}$, have been shown to be a respiratory concern despite the each facility's remote location [39–41]. LADWP is aggressively pursuing divestiture in its 21% share of NGS and 100% share of IPP which will lead to significant long-term benefits for the Gold LRT [31].

Figure 1 shows that significant environmental benefits can be achieved by automobiles, Orange BRT, and Gold LRT in the long-term as a result of established energy and environmental policies as well as vehicle technology changes, and that public transit technology and energy changes will produce more environmental benefits per trip than automobiles. In the near-term, both the Orange BRT and Gold LRT lines can be expected to achieve lower energy and GHG impacts per PMT than emerging 35 mile gallon^{-1} automobiles. While propulsion effects (vehicle operation and propulsion electricity) constitute a majority share of life-cycle effects for energy and GHGs, vehicle manufacturing, energy production, and in the case of the Gold line, electricity for infrastructure operation (train control, lighting, stations, etc) contribute significantly. Due to high NO_x and $PM_{2.5}$ emissions in coal-fired electricity generation, Gold LRT in the near-term creates large potential smog and respiratory impacts, however, the replacement of this coal electricity with natural gas by 2015–2025 will result in significant reductions in the long-term [31]. For non-GHG air emissions, indirect and supply chain processes (in this case vehicle manufacturing and infrastructure construction) typically dominate the life-cycle footprint of modes showing how vast supply chains that traverse geopolitical boundaries result in remote impacts far from where the decision to build and operate a transportation mode occurs. Diesel equipment use, material processing, and electricity generation for the production and distribution of materials throughout the supply chain generate heavy NO_x and $PM_{2.5}$

emissions that when allocated to LA travel can dominate the life-cycle smog and respiratory effects.

In the long-term, automobile fuel economy gains, reduced emission buses, and RPS electricity will have the greatest impacts on passenger transportation energy use and GHG emissions in LA. Larger renewable shares feeding Orange BRT bus manufacturing drives a 46% reduction in life-cycle respiratory impacts. For the Gold LRT, RPS electricity will reduce both propulsion and infrastructure operation smog effects by 93%. Automobile indirect effects show non-negligible contributions to life-cycle impacts when allocated across all trip takers. The impacts of station access and egress by motorized travel are explored in later sections.

LCA transcends geopolitical boundaries in its assessment of indirect and supply chain processes, and urban sustainability policy makers should recognize that local vehicle travel triggers energy use and emissions outside of cities. This is clear for coal-fired electricity generation in Arizona but can become complex when moving up the supply chain for vehicle and infrastructure components. Vehicle operation and propulsion electricity effects are a large portion of energy consumption and GHG emissions and will occur locally while energy production (i.e., primary fuel extraction and processing) and vehicle manufacturing occur remotely. For the sedan, roughly 72–77% of life-cycle energy consumption and GHG emissions occurs locally meaning that for every 75 MJ of energy consumed or grams of CO_{2e} emitted in LA, an additional 25 are triggered outside of the city. For the Orange BRT, local energy use and GHG emissions constitute 74–82% and for the Gold LRT, only 53–62% due to electricity generation both outside of the county and the state. These percentages change significantly for smog and respiratory stressors due to the larger contributions of non-propulsion effects in the life-cycle.

For the sedan, remote electricity generation for vehicle manufacturing and energy production emissions mean that only 52–73% of potential impacts may occur locally. Similarly, remote vehicle manufacturing and CNG production emissions for the Orange BRT result in roughly 55–76% of respiratory impact stressors occurring locally. Due to out-of-state coal electricity generation, in the near-term the Gold LRT line has the lowest fraction of life-cycle smog and respiratory effects occurring locally, at 54% and 31%. Urban energy and environmental goals should recognize

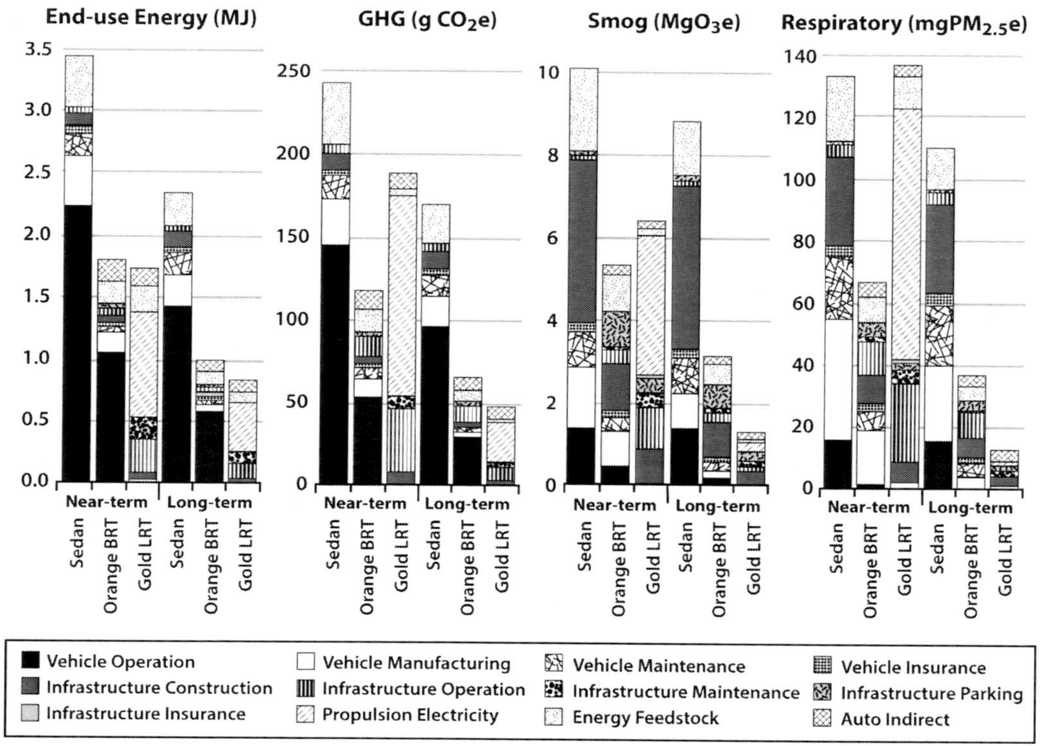

Figure 1. Life-cycle per PMT results for average occupancy vehicles. For each impact both near-term and long-term results are shown for each mode. Vehicle tailpipe effects are gray, vehicle are blue, infrastructure are red, and energy production are green. Local impacts are shown with a line on the left of the life-cycle result and remote on the right if the dominating share of effects occurs inside or outside of LA county.

that cities rely on complex and dynamic energy and material supply chain networks and that it may be possible through contracts or supplier selection to reduce remote impacts. This will only occur if policymakers adopt an environmental assessment framework that acknowledges that cities are not isolated systems and trigger resource use and emissions that exist beyond their geopolitical boundaries [42].

The per PMT assessment is valuable for understanding how regions should allocate their total emissions or impacts to each mode's travel and identify which life-cycle processes should be targeted for the greatest environmental gains, however, a consequential assessment is needed for assessing how new modes will contribute to a city reaching their environmental goals, by comparing against a regional baseline.

4.4 PUBLIC TRANSIT FOR ENERGY AND ENVIRONMENTAL GOALS

To assess the effects of the decision to deploy a public transit system and how such a system contributes to a city reaching an environmental goal, a consequential LCA framework must be used. The decision to deploy the Orange and Gold lines resulted in the operation of new vehicles that require infrastructure and trigger life-cycle processes that consume energy and generate emissions. While induced demand is created, reduced automobile travel has also occurred [9, 33], which should reduce future energy consumption and emissions from personal vehicles. A consequential LCA is used to assess the increased impacts from new transit modes and avoided impacts of reduced automobile travel. Future adoption forecasts [5] are used with mode shift survey results to develop the decadal benefit–cost impact assessment and payback estimates shown in figure 2.

For both transit lines, construction impacts (light red life-cycle bar) begin the series in the first decade. Starting in the second decade the transit systems begin operation, offsetting automobile travel, and over the coming decades reach ridership maturity. For both modes and all impacts, the benefits from reduced automobile travel outweigh the environmental costs of the new transit systems. The avoided impacts are 1.5–3 times larger for GHG emissions than the added transit emissions, 1.3–5.5 times for smog,

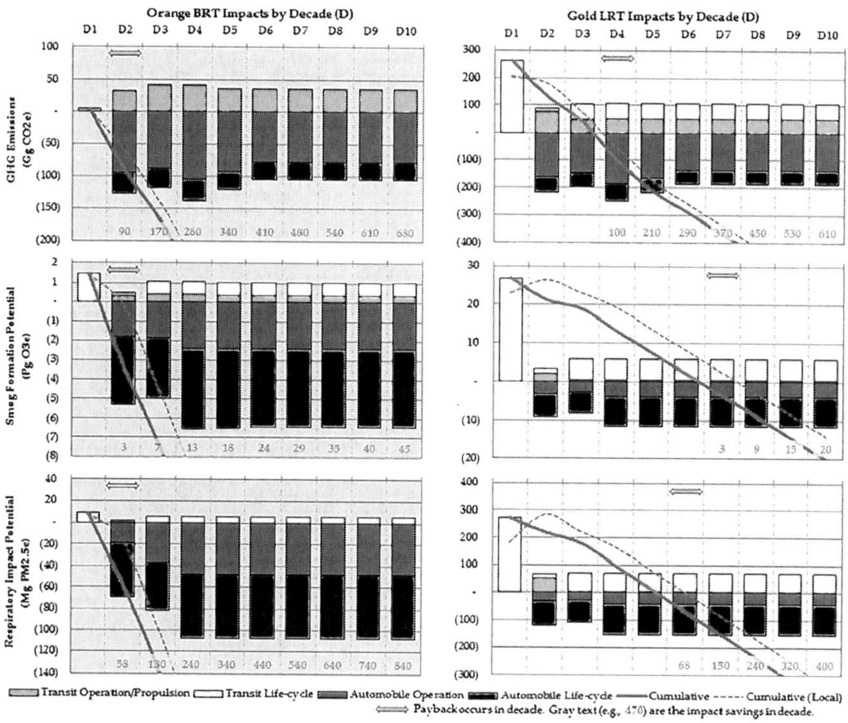

Figure 2. Environmental impact schedules and resulting paybacks. Decadal (D) life-cycle results (bars) are shown for the new transit system (red) and avoided automobile (blue) effects. Cumulative (i.e., net effects) life-cycle and local green lines are shown and when they cross the abscissae have resulted in a net reduction of impacts as a result of the transit system. When payback occurs, the net benefits are shown at the bottom of the decade.

and 1.4–15 times for respiratory impacts. There are significantly fewer impacts produced from the initial construction of the dedicated Orange BRT right-of-way than from the Gold LRT tracks due to a variety of process, material, and supply chain life-cycle effects. The heavy use of concrete for Gold line tracks results in significant CO_2, VOC, and $PM_{2.5}$ releases during cement and concrete production due to calcination of limestone and emissions of organics elements and fine particles during kiln firing. The result is that the Orange line payback for GHGs and respiratory effects

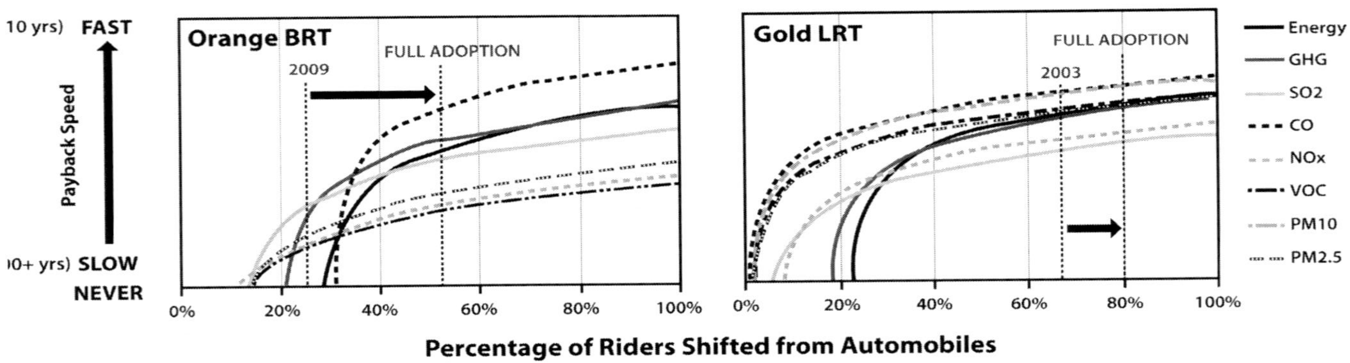

Figure 3. Transit energy and environmental payback speed with automobile shifts. The different payback speed curves are shown as a function of the percentage of transit riders having shifted from automobiles. For each mode, current and forecasted full adoption levels are shown as dashed vertical gray lines. At the abscissa, payback does not occur.

is almost immediate and the Gold line paybacks occur 30–60 years after operation begins. The results highlight the sensitivity of payback to auto trips shifted to transit. Transportation planners can position new transit to help cities meet environmental goals by developing strategies that ensure certain levels of automobile shifting are achieved to accelerate paybacks. Figure 3 shows the payback speed for energy consumption and air emissions as a response to the percentage of transit trip takers that have shifted from automobiles.

Figure 3 shows that with greater shifts to transit from automobiles paybacks occur more quickly. This response will hold true for any public transit system where the per PMT effects of automobiles are larger than the public transit mode. The life-cycle energy and emissions curves have different intercepts and trajectories showing that paybacks will occur at different rates, and will not be the same for any environmental indicator. A transit system that achieves 50% of riders having shifted from automobiles will experience a different payback date for VOCs than it will for GHGs. The Orange line's 2009 25% shift is currently below the 30% needed to produce energy and CO reductions, however, given the anticipated full adoption shift of 52% the system will over 50 years produce a net reduction of 320 Gg CO_{2e} (see figure 2). The information in figure 3, while specific to the LA transit systems, can provide valuable goals for cities. For any mode, there is a minimum window of percentage of transit riders shifted from automobiles where pollutants will be reduced. For example, the abscissa for the Orange BRT reveals that at between roughly 10% and 30% pollutant reductions will be achieved (how quickly is a separate question). At 30%, the Orange BRT system is guaranteed to have payback across all pollutants. This maximum in the window can be used by cities that are discussing the implementation of new transit systems to help meet environmental goals. Planning efforts should be coordinated such that the systems achieve these minimum mode shifts.

4.5 DOOR-TO-DOOR LIFE-CYCLE EFFECTS

Transportation environmental policies should consider the multi-modal door-to-door impacts of trips, and LCA can provide valuable insight for both the operational and non-operational effects of a traveler's choice. A life-cycle understanding of door-to-door trips is particularly important for transit travelers whose access or egress to stations occurs by automobile where questions arise of the benefits of these trips, particularly when infrastructure (specifically station parking) is included. A door-to-door GHG LCA is developed for a unimodal automobile trip compared against each transit line. For each transit line, access/egress is shown with local bus service as well as by automobile. Typical trip distances are used (as described in previous sections) and processing of LA Metro and travel survey data provides information on feeder bus and automobile typical trip characteristics [7, 8, 32, 33]. The typical Orange BRT trip is 6 mile with feeder bus and auto trips adding on average 1.8 and 4.2 mile respectively. A competing unimodal auto trip is 10.2 mile assuming distance shifts identified in the previously described mode shift clustering analysis [7, 32]. The typical Gold LRT trip is 7.5 mile with feeder bus and auto trips of 3.3 and 5 mile and is compared against a 12.5 mile competing auto trip [7, 32, 33]. Current and future Orange BRT, Gold LRT, and feeder bus offpeak, average, and peak occupancies are determined from LA Metro data and forecasts [5, 7]. Auto feeder travel is shown as both average and single occupancy travel. The impacts of the 4 700 and 2 300 parking spaces (shown as bright orange in figure 1) are now shifted to the automobile feeder trips. The results are shown in figure 4 in both the near-term and long-term for GHG emissions for offpeak, average, and peak travel.

The Orange BRT and Gold LRT door-to-door trips with typical access/egress by other local buses or automobiles are likely to have a lower life-cycle footprint than a competing unimodal automobile trip. The only exceptions are offpeak (low occupancy) transit travel with single occupancy automobile feeder access/egress compared against average (1.7 passenger) unimodal auto trips. Transit travel (even with single occupancy automobile feeder access/egress) consistently produces lower impacts than a competing single occupancy automobile trip. On average, transit+local bus trips have 77% lower GHG trip footprints than a competing automobile trip and transit+auto 52% lower. Recent onboard travel surveys report that 49% of Orange BRT passengers arrive to or leave from stations by local transit and 14% by automobile, and for the Gold line 41% link bus and other rail trips (data on access/egress by automobile were not identified)

[9, 33]. Strategies that shift travelers from automobiles to public transit-only service produces the greatest environmental benefits and parking infrastructure management is central to changing behavior [43]. Figure 4 shows that parking construction and maintenance (orange bar) impacts for transit+auto trips can be as large as the transit infrastructure construction and maintenance (pink bars) per trip. These infrastructure enable the emergent travel behavior and the provision of low cost or free parking at LA Metro stations helps to encourage the auto access/egress impacts [43]. Environmental benefit–cost analyses should consider the life-cycle tradeoffs of land use for station parking versus transit-oriented development (TOD) and the co-benefits that could be achieved by TODs in reducing both auto access/egress impacts and household energy use [44].

4.6 INTEGRATING TRANSPORTATION LCA IN URBAN ENVIRONMENTAL POLICYMAKING

Public transit systems are typically positioned as transportation environmental impact reducers and as policy and decision makers begin to incorporate life-cycle thinking into planning, new strategies must be developed for integrating LCA. The results show that both local and remote life-cycle environmental impacts will be reduced by implementing BRT and LRT for all impacts in the long-term. The results also show that the decision to implement a new transit system in a city has significant local and remote energy and environmental impacts beyond vehicle operation. These life-cycle impacts are the result of indirect and supply chain processes that are often ignored by policy and decision makers, as well as environmental mitigation strategies.

Challenges exist for implementing life-cycle results in governmental processes [45]. Because life-cycle emissions are distributed across numerous air basins throughout the United States and the world, there exists a spatial mismatch for policymaking. Both transportation planning and emissions control policy structures in the United States are fragmented across jurisdictions and across different components of the life-cycle. The transportation system is created through a series of federal, state, regional and local programs and authorities acting in an independent, yet interde-

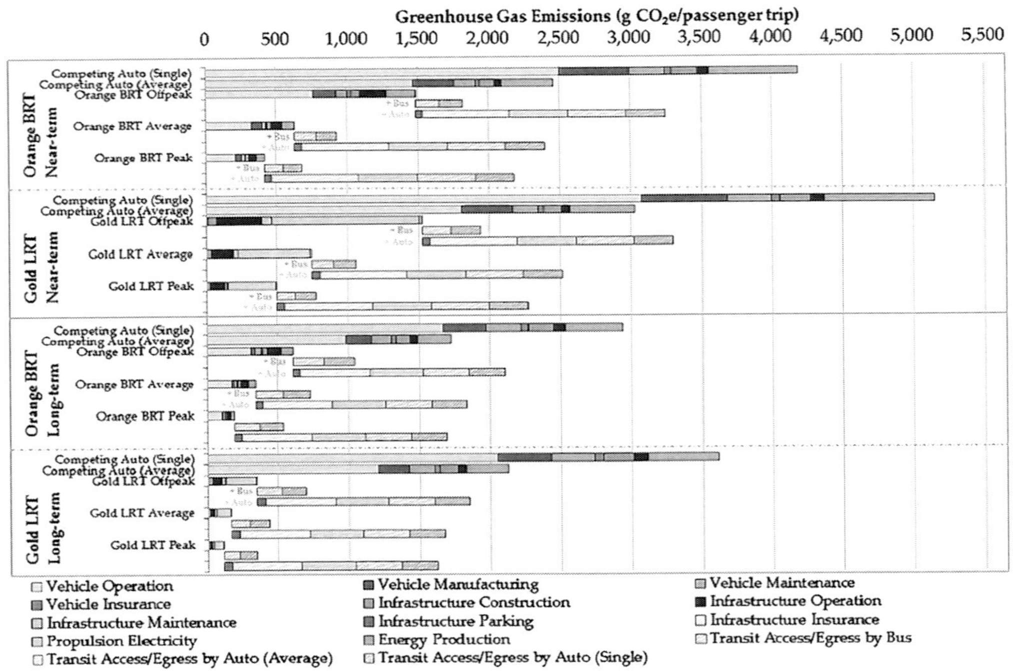

Figure 4. Life-cycle door-to-door ghg comparison. For the transit modes, feeder bus and automobile impacts should be assessed cumulatively. For example, an Orange BRT or Gold LRT trip that starts or ends with a bus trip is equal to the transit life-cycle bar plus the bus purple striped bars. Feeder bus and auto travel results are shown with both operational (striped bar with white background) and life-cycle (striped bar with gray background) portions. For auto access/egress to transit, the effects of average occupancy (1.7) passengers per car is shown as orange stripes and if the automobile was single occupancy then the red striped bar would be added on. Bike and walk impacts are not considered.

pendent, manner. Designing a policy structure to reduce life-cycle emissions is therefore a complex task, and a variety of policy options may be viable. While there is no simple policy fix, mitigation strategies that effectively incorporate LCA into transportation planning should involve all of the following:

i. changing analytical and decision criteria for project selection;
ii. improving the capability to compare different trans- portation modes to one another in planning and project financing processes;
iii. improving the capability to conduct analysis of complex environmental impacts into transportation planning before project selection occurs (i.e. not only in post-decisional environmental impact assessments);
iv. improving analytical integration across different spatial and temporal scales; and,
v. creating purchasing strategies that emphasize the use of products and materials with higher recycled content and establish relationships with suppliers that have instituted efficiency measures.

Given these needs, the metropolitan region is likely the most useful geographic scale for transportation LCA integration and LCA can be used as a valuable guiding framework for novel mitigation strategies. Metropolitan Planning Organizations (MPOs) already offer the greatest planning integration across modes and already possess relatively advanced analytical and planning capabilities for the development of Regional Transportation Plans. Pigovian tax or cap-and-trade structures for carbon or other emissions can use life-cycle results to capture indirect and supply chain impacts and if cast at a large geographic scale can reduce urban and hinterland impacts by transcending the notion that activities in cities are contained within a geopolitical boundary.

REFERENCES

1. CARB 2011 California Greenhouse Gas Emissions Inventory: 2000–2009 (Sacramento, CA: California Air Resources Board)

2. Ostro Betal 2007 The effects of components offine particulate air pollution on mortality in California: results from CALFINE Environ. Health Perspect. 115 13–9
3. Chester M and Horvath A 2009 Environmental assessmentof passenger transportation should include infrastructure and supply chains Environ. Res. Lett. 4 024008
4. Chester M and Horvath A 2012 High-speed rail with emerging automobiles and aircraft can reduce environmental impacts in California's future Environ. Res. Lett. 7 034012
5. LA Metro 2012 Personal Communications with Los Angeles County Metropolitan Transportation Authority: Emmanuel Liban (2011–2012), John Drayton (July 15, 2011), Alvin Kusumoto (August 2, 2011), Scott Page (August 2, 2011), James Jimenez (July 26, 2011), and Susan Phifer (Planning Manager, August 3, 2011) (Los Angeles, CA: Los Angeles County Metropolitan Transportation Authority)
6. Chester M et al 2012 Environmental Life-Cycle Assessment of Los Angeles Metro's Orange Bus Rapid Transit and Gold Light Rail Transit Lines (Arizona State University Report No. SSEBE-CESEM-2012-WPS-003) (Tempe, AZ: Arizona State University)
7. LA Metro 2011 Bu sand Rail Ridership Estimates and Passenger Overview (Los Angeles, CA: Los Angeles Metropolitan Transportation Authority)
8. LA Metro 2011 Metro Orange Line Mode Shift Study and Greenhouse Gas Emissions Analysis (Los Angeles, CA: Los Angeles Metropolitan Transportation Authority)
9. Flynn J et al 2011 Metro Orange Line BRT Project Evaluation (Washington, DC: Federal Transit Administration)
10. City of LA 2012 Final Program Environmental Impact Report for the Warner Center Regional Core Comprehensive Specific Plan (Los Angeles, CA: City of Los Angeles)
11. US Energy Information Administration 2012 Annual Energy Outlook (Washington, DC: US Department of Energy)
12. EEA 2010 National Renewable Energy Action Plan Data from Member States (Copenhagen: European Environment Agency)
13. SimaPro 2012 SimaPro v7.3.3 Using the Ecoinvent v2.2 Database (Amersfoort: PRe´ Consultants)
14. GREET 2012 Greenhouse Gases, Regulated Emissions, and Energy Use in Transportation (GREET; 1: Fuel Cycle; 2: Vehicle Cycle) Model (Argonne, IL: Argonne National Laboratory)
15. PaLATE 2004 Pavement Life-cycle Assessment for Environmental and Economic Effects (Berkeley, CA: University of California)
16. LA Metro 2000 San Fernando Valley East–West Transit Corridor, Major Investment Study (Los Angeles, CA: Los Angeles Metropolitan Transportation Authority)
17. CARB 2000 Risk Reduction Plan to Reduce Particulate Matter Emissions from Diesel-Fueled Engines and Vehicles (Sacramento, CA: California Air Resources Board)
18. Gautam Metal 2011 Testing of Volatile and Nonvolatile Emissions for Advanced Technology Natural Gas Vehicles (Morgantown, WV: West Virginia University)
19. Ayala A et al 2003 Oxidation catalys teffect on CNG transit bus emissions Technical Report (Warrendale, PA: Society of Automotive Engineers) doi:10.4271/2003-01-1900
20. Ayala A et al 2002 Diese land CNG heavy-dutytransitbus emissions over multiple driving schedules: regulated pollutants and project overview Technical Report (Warrendale, PA: Society of Automotive Engineers) doi:10.4271/2002-01-1722

21. NREL 2006 Washington Metropolitan Area Transit Authority: Compressed Natural Gas Transit Bus Evaluation (Golden, CO: National Renewable Energy Laboratory)
22. NREL 2005 Emission Testing of Washington Metropolitan Area Transit Authority (WMATA) Natural Gas and Diesel Transit Buses (Golden, CO: National Renewable Energy Laboratory)
23. Kado N et al2005Emissionsoftoxicpollutantsfrom compressed natural gas and low sulfur diesel-fueled heavy-duty transit buses tested over multiple driving cycles Environ. Sci. Technol. 39 7638–49
24. LanniTetal2003Performanceandemissionsevaluationof compressed natural gas and clean diesel buses at New York city's Metropolitan transit authority Technical Report (Warrendale, PA: Society of Automotive Engineers) doi:10.4271/2003-01-0300
25. Clark N et al 1999 Diesel and CNG transit bus emissions characterizaion by two chassis dynamometer laboratories: results and issues Technical Report (Warrendale, PA: Society of Automotive Engineers) doi:10.4271/1999-01- 1469
26. Nylund N-O et al 2004 Transit Bus Emission Study: Comparison of Emissions from Diesel and Natural Gas Buses (Finland: VTT)
27. Ayala A et al 2003 CNG and diesel transit bus emissions in review 9th Diesel Engine Emissions Reduction Conference (Newport, RI: US EPA)
28. ICCT 2009 CNG Bus Emissions Roadmap: From Euro III to Euro VI (Washington, DC: The International Council on Clean Transportation)
29. LACTC 1988 Draft Environmental Impact Report for the Pasadena–Los Angeles Rail Transit Project (Los Angeles, CA: Los Angeles County Transportation Commission)
30. USDOT 2009 National Transit Database (Washington, DC: US Department of Transportation)
31. LA DWP 2011 Power Integrated Resource Plan (Los Angeles, CA: Los Angeles Department of Water and Power)
32. NHTS 2009 National Household Travel Survey (Oak Ridge, TN: US Department of Transportation's Oak Ridge National Laboratory)
33. LA Metro 2004 Gold Line Corridor Before/After Study Combined Report (Los Angeles, CA: Los Angeles Metropolitan Transportation Authority)
34. USDOT 2012 National Transportation Statistics (Washington, DC: US Department of Transportation)
35. LA Metro 2012 Sepulveda Pass Corridor Systems Planning Study (Los Angeles, CA: Los Angeles County Metropolitan Transportation Authority)
36. Fraley C and Raftery AE 2002 Model-based clustering, discriminant analysis, and density estimation J. Am. Stat. Assoc. 97 611–31
37. Bare JC 2002 TRACI: the tool for the reduction and assessment of chemical and other environmental impacts J. Indust. Ecol. 6 49–78
38. EPA 2013 Joint Federal Agency Statement Regarding Navajo Generating Station (Washington, DC: US Environmental Protection Agency)
39. GAO 2012 Air Emissions and Electricity Generationat US Power Plants (Washington, DC: US Government Accountability Office)
40. Eatough DJ et al 1996 Apportionment of sulfuroxides at canyonlands during the winter of 1990—I. Study design and particulate chemical composition Atmos. Environ. 30 269–81

41. Wilson JC and McMurry PH 1981 Studies of aerosol formation in power plant plumes—II. Secondary aerosol formation in the Navajo generating station plume Atmos. Environ. 15 2329–39
42. Chester M, Pincetl S and Allenby B 2012 Avoiding unintended tradeoffs by integrating life-cycle impact assessment with urban metabolism Curr. Opin. Environ. Sustain. 4 451–7
43. Shoup D 2011 The High Cost of Free Parking (Chicago, IL: American Planning Association)
44. Kimball M et al 2012 Policy Brief: Transit-Oriented Development Infill in Phoenix can Reduce Future Transportation and Land Use Life-Cycle Environmental Impacts (Arizona State University Report No. SSEBE-CESEM-2012-RPR-002) (Tempe, AZ: Arizona State University)
45. Eisenstein W, Chester M and Pincetl S2013 Policy options for incorporating life-cycle environmental assessment into transportation planning Transp. Res. Rec. at press

There are results data that are not available in this version of the article. To view this additional information, please go to www.transportationlca.org.

CHAPTER 5

Recent Photocatalytic Applications for Air Purification in Belgium

ELIA BOONEN AND ANNE BEELDENS

5.1 INTRODUCTION

Emission from the transport sector has a particular impact on the overall air quality because of its rapid rate of growth: goods transport by road in Europe (EU-27) has increased by 31% (period 1995–2009), while passenger transport by road in the EU-27 has gone up by 21% and passenger transport in air by 51% in the same period [1]. The main emissions caused by motor traffic are nitrogen oxides (NO_x), hydrocarbons (HC) and carbon monoxide (CO), accounting for respectively 46%, 50% and 36% of all such emissions in Europe in 2008 [2].

These pollutants have an increasing impact on the urban air quality. In addition, photochemical reactions resulting from the action of sunlight on NO_2 and VOC's (volatile organic compounds) lead to the formation of "photochemical smog" and ozone, a secondary long-range pollutant, which impacts in rural areas often far from the original emission site. Acid rain is another long-range pollutant influenced by vehicle NO_x emissions and resulting from the transport of NO_x, oxidation in the air into HNO_3 and finally, precipitation of (acid) NO_3^- with harmful consequences for building materials (corrosion of the surface) and vegetation.

The European Directives [3] impose a limit to the NO_2 concentration in ambient air of maximum 40 μg/m³ NO_2 (21 ppbV) averaged over 1 year and 200 μg/m³ (106 ppbV) averaged over 1 h. These limit values gradually decreased from 50 and 250 in 2005 to the final limit in 2010.

Heterogeneous photocatalysis is a promising method for NO_x abatement. In the presence of UV-light, the photocatalytically active form of TiO_2 present at the surface of the material is activated, enabling the abatement of pollutants in the air. The translation from laboratory results to real cases is starting. Different applications are implemented in Belgium in order to see the influence of the photocatalytic materials on real scale and to determine the durability of the air purifying capacity over time.

In the first part of this paper, the principle of photocatalytic concrete will be elaborated, followed by a description of the past laboratory research indicating important influencing factors for the purifying process. Next, an overview of the results regarding the first pilot project in Antwerp [2] is given, and finally, the different applications in Belgium that have recently been finished, will be discussed.

5.2 PHOTOCATALYTIC CONCRETE: PURIFYING THE AIR THROUGH THE PAVEMENT

A solution for the air pollution by traffic can be found in the treatment of the pollutants as close to the source as possible. Therefore, photocatalytically active materials can be added to the surface of pavement and building materials [4]. Air purification through heterogeneous photocatalysis consists of different steps: under the influence of UV-light, the photoactive TiO_2 at the surface of the material is activated. Subsequently, the pollutants are oxidized due to the presence of the photocatalyst and precipitated on the surface of the material. Finally, they can be removed from the surface by the rain or cleaning/washing with water, see Figure 1.

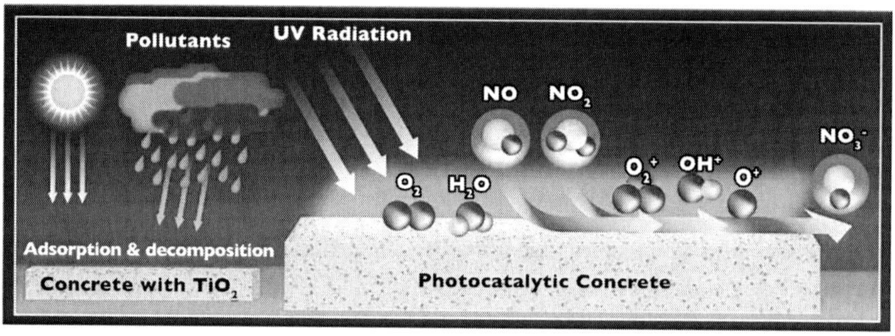

Figure 1. Schematic of photocatalytic air purifying pavement.

Heterogeneous photocatalysis with titanium dioxide (TiO_2) as catalyst is a rapidly developing field in environmental engineering, as it has a great potential to cope with the increasing pollution. Besides its self-cleaning properties, it is known since almost 100 years that titanium dioxide acts as a photo-catalyst that can decompose pollutants under UV radiation [5]. The impulse for the more widespread use of TiO_2 photocatalytic materials was further given in 1972 by Fujishima and Honda [6], who discovered the hydrolysis of water in the presence of light, by means of a TiO_2-anode in a photochemical cell. In the 1980s, organic pollution in water was also decomposed by adding TiO_2 and under influence of UV-light [7]. The application of TiO_2, in the photo-active crystalline phase anatase, as air purifying material originated in Japan in 1996 (e.g., [8]). Since then, a broad spectrum of products appeared on the market for indoor use as well as for outdoor applications. Regarding traffic emissions, it is important that the exhaust gases stay in contact with the active surface during a certain period. The street configuration, the speed of the traffic, the speed and direction of the wind, all influence the final reduction rate of pollutants in situ.

In the case of concrete pavement blocks [9,10], the anatase is added to the wearing layer of the pavers which is approximately 8 mm thick. In the case of cast-in-place concrete pavements, the TiO_2 is added in the top layer (40 mm thick). The fact that the TiO_2 is present over the whole thickness of this layer means that even if some surface wear takes place, for example by traffic or weathering, new TiO_2 will be present at the surface to maintain the photocatalytic activity (in contrast to the abrasion of a coating or dispersion layer for instance). The use of TiO_2 in combination with cement leads to a transformation of the NO_x into NO_3^-, which is adsorbed at the surface due to the alkalinity of the concrete [11]. Thus, a synergetic effect is created in the presence of the cement matrix, which helps to effectively trap the reactant gases (NO and NO_2) together with the nitrate salt formed. Subsequently, the deposited nitrate can be washed away by rain or washing with water. In addition, these nitrates pose no real threat towards pollution of body waters because the resulting concentrations in the waste water are very low, even below the current limit values for surface and ground water [12].

Special attention is given here to the NO and NO_2 content in the air, since they are for almost 50% caused by the exhaust of traffic and are at the base of smog, secondary ozone and acid rain formation as indicated above. The photocatalytic oxidation of NO is usually assumed to be a surface reaction between NO and an oxidizing species formed upon the adsorption of a photon by the photocatalyst, e.g., a hydroxyl radical, both adsorbed at the surface of the photocatalyst [13]. It has been shown by various authors that the final product of the photocatalytic oxidation of NO in the presence of TiO_2 is nitric acid (HNO_3) while HNO_2 and NO_2 have been identified as intermediate products in the gas phase over the photocatalyst [2,4,11,13,14]. The resulting reaction pathway of the photocatalytic oxidation of NO has been discussed in several publications e.g., [2,4,13–16] most of which proposed the photocatalytic conversion of NO via HNO_2 to yield NO_2, which is subsequently oxidized by the attack of a hydroxyl radical to the final product HNO_3:

$$NO_{ads} + OH_{ads} \rightarrow HNO_{2ads}$$

$$HNO_{2ads} + OH_{ads} \rightarrow NO_{2ads} + H_2O_{ads}$$

$$NO_{2ads} + OH_{ads} \rightarrow HNO_{3ads}$$

Here, all nitrogen compounds adsorbed at the photocatalyst surface are assumed to be in equilibrium with the gas phase.

Until now, UV-light (in the UV-A spectrum) was necessary to activate the photocatalyst. However, recent research indicates a shift towards the visible light [17], for instance by doping the TiO_2 with transition metal ions or non-metallic anionic species, or forming reduced TiO_x. These techniques introduce impurities and defects in the band gap of TiO_2 thereby increasing the amount of visible light that can be absorbed and used in the photocatalytic process. This means that applications in tunnels and indoor environments become more realistic. Especially the application in tunnels is worth looking at due to the high concentration of air pollutants at these sites. One of the projects in Belgium is focusing on this subject [18].

5.3 LABORATORY RESULTS: PARAMETER EVALUATION

Different test methods have been developed to determine the efficiency of photocatalytic materials towards air purification. An overview is given in [11]. A distinction can be made by the type of air flow; in the flow-through method according to ISO 22197-1 [19], the air, with a concentration of 1 ppmV of NO, passes once-only over the sample which is illuminated by a UV-lamp with light intensity equal to 10 W/m^2 in the range between 300 and 400 nm, as illustrated in Figure 2. Afterwards, the NO_x (= sum of NO and NO_2) concentration is measured at the outlet and the reduction (in %) is calculated. It is also worth to note here that within Europe actions are underway to harmonize and develop new standards for photocatalyis [20]. In any case, the test procedure used for the current results is still based on the existing ISO standard.

The pre-treatment of the samples in the laboratory can be important to obtain reproducible results and mainly depends on the type of base material (e.g., concrete or paints). A typical test scheme according to the ISO standard is presented in Figure 3, where the following steps are applied to the sample: 0.5 h at 1 ppmV NO concentration, no light—5 h exposure to an air flow of 3 L/min with 1 ppmV NO and UV-illumination—0.5 h with UV-illumination and no exposure. A small increase with time of the NOx concentration is visible due to the deposit of the NO_3^- at the surface.

The influence of different important test parameters affecting the photocatalytic reaction has been investigated before [2] such as temperature, light intensity, relative humidity, contact time (controlled by surface area, flow velocity, height of air flow, etc.). For instance, the effect of relative humidity of the ingoing air is illustrated in Figure 4 for different materials including cementitious (concrete, mortar) and other (paint) substrates. Clearly, for cementitious materials the reduction of the NO_x concentration in the outlet air decreases with increasing relative humidity (RH, %), an observation which was also found by other authors [21]. This probably has to do with the fact that the water in the atmosphere plays a role in the adhesion of the pollutants at the surface and with the competition effect that can arise between water molecules and NO_x in the ambient air with increasing RH. For paints (acidic environment) though, it has been noticed that there is an optimum in RH where a maximal efficiency is obtained. Anyway, relative humidity proves to be an important limiting factor for photocatalytic applications in humid areas like Belgium. Temperature on the other hand, was found to have no significant influence on the NO_x reduction within the ambient range (5–25 °C).

In general, it can be stated that the efficiency towards the reduction of NO_x (in %) increases with a longer contact time (larger surface area, lower air velocity, smaller height of air flow, higher turbulence at the surface), a lower relative humidity (for cementitious materials) and a higher intensity of incident light. These are the conditions at which the risk of ozone formation in summer is the largest: higher sun light intensity, no wind and no rain. At these days, the photocatalytic reaction will be more pronounced.

5.4 PILOT PROJECT IN ANTWERP

An important issue is the conversion of the results obtained in the laboratory to real applications. In order to see the influence of photocatalytic pavements in "real conditions", a first pilot section of 10.000 m^2 of photocatalytic pavement blocks was constructed in 2004–2005 on the parking lanes of a main axe in Antwerp [2]. Figure 5 depicts a view of the parking lane, where the photocatalytic concrete pavement blocks have been applied. Only the wearing layer (upper 5–6 mm) of the blocks contains ana-

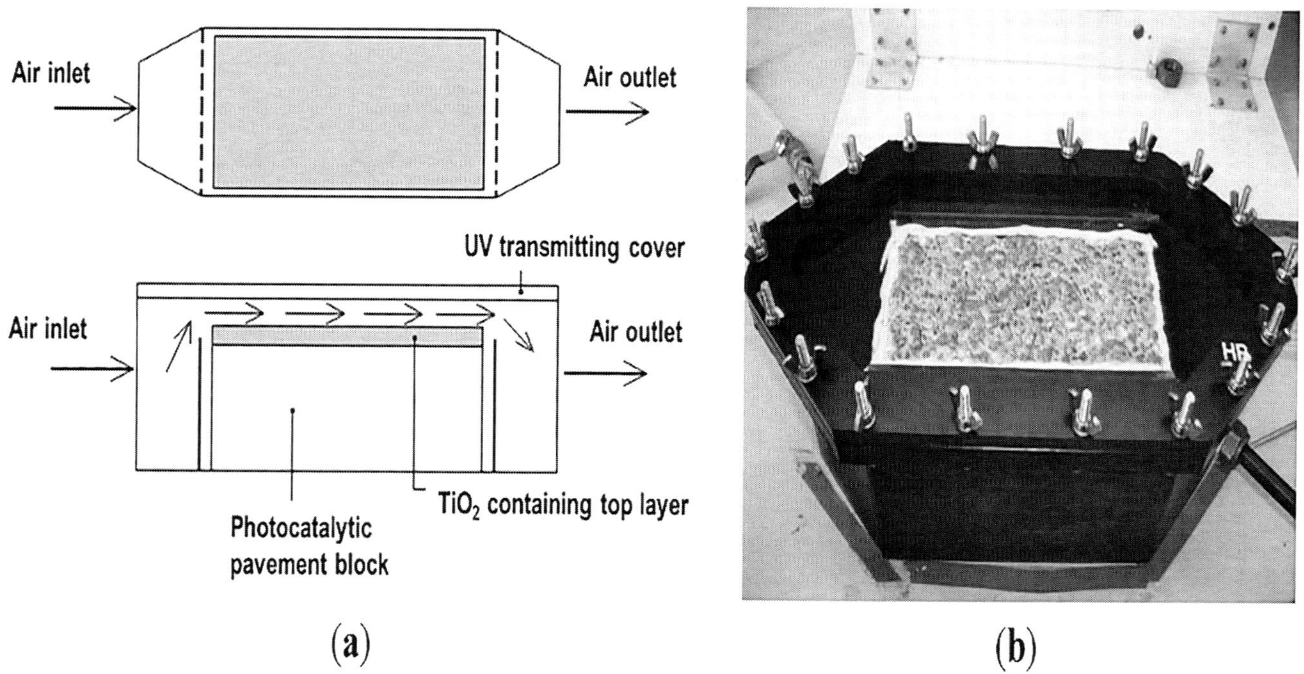

Figure 2. (a) Schematic and (b) photo of measurement set-up based on ISO 22197-1:2007 [19] at Belgian Road Research Center (BRRC).

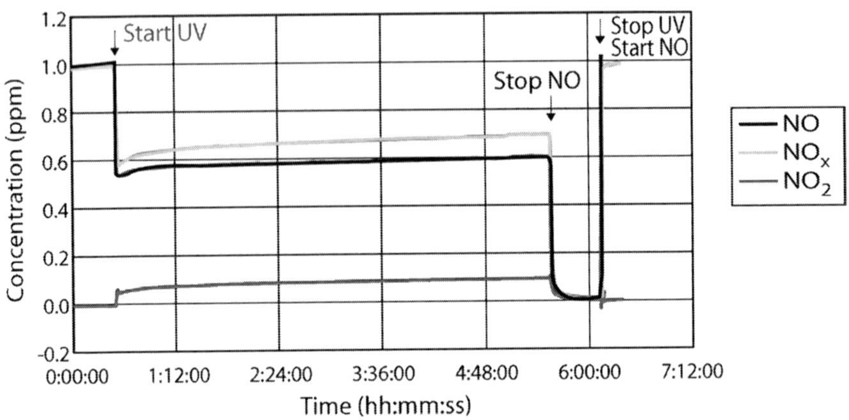

Figure 3. Typical result obtained in the laboratory following the standard ISO test procedure.

tase TiO_2 mixed in the mass of the concrete layer. The exact composition could not be given by the manufacturer (Marlux, Tessenderlo, Belgium) at that time in view of confidentiality. In spite of the fact that the surface applied on the Leien of Antwerp is quite important, one has to notice the relatively small width of the photocatalytic parking lanes in comparison with the total street: 2 × 4.5 m versus a total width of 60 m.

In order to check the durability of the photocatalytic efficiency, pavement blocks were taken from the lane after different periods of exposure and measured in the laboratory with and without washing of the surface. Some of the results are presented in Figure 6. They indicate a good durability of the efficiency towards NO_x abatement. The deposition of pollutants on the surface leads to a decrease in efficiency which can be regained after washing. Recently repeated measurements in 2010 indicate that even after more than five years of service life, the photocatalytic efficiency of the pavers is still present [22].

Besides the tests in the lab, on site measurements were also carried out. Since no reference measurements without photocatalytic material (prior to the application) exist, the interpretation of these results is rather difficult. Especially the influence of traffic, wind speed, light intensity and relative

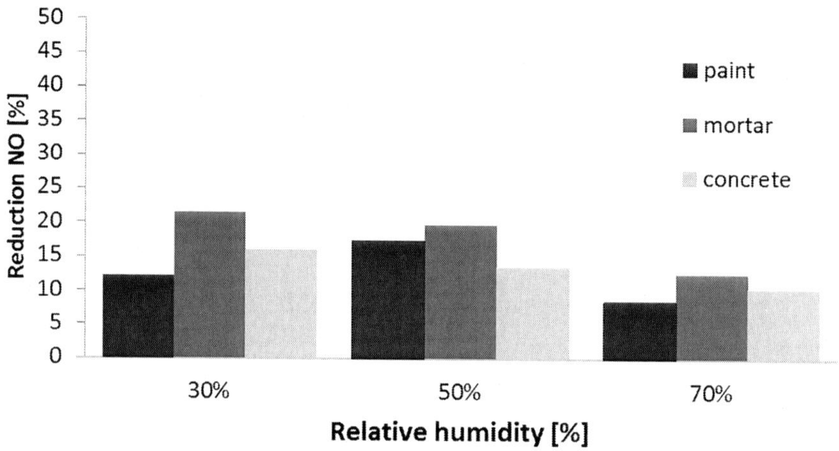

Figure 4. Effect of relative humidity on photocatalytic efficiency for different materials.

humidity are playing an important role. Detailed results can be found in [2]. In brief, the field measurements suggested a decrease in NO_x concentration at the sites with photocatalytic materials, where a levelling out of the pollution peaks is visible. In any case, precaution has to be taken with the interpretation of data since these results are momentary and limited over time. However, at least, they gave an indication of the efficiency of the photocatalytic pavement materials in situ, and a basis to work on for future applications.

5.5 RECENT PHOTOCATALYTIC APPLICATIONS IN BELGIUM

Since the first application in Antwerp (2004–2005), much progress has been made within the photocatalytic research area. Newer, better and more efficient materials are constantly being developed, and action is more and more broadened also to visible light responsive materials [17]. This also

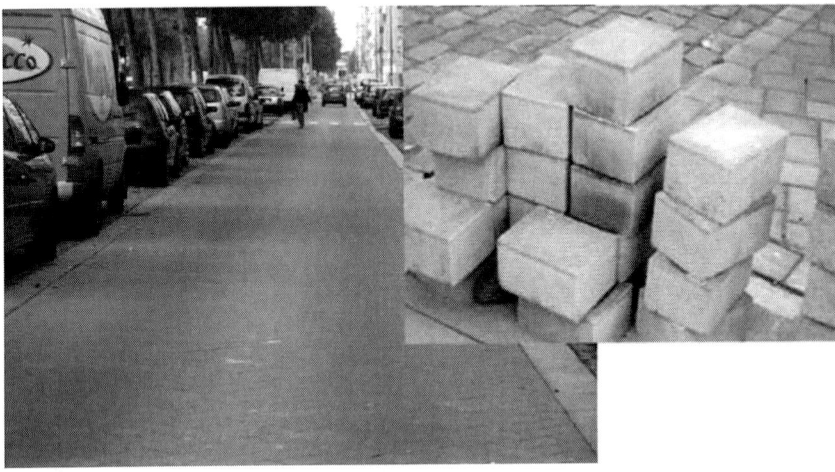

Figure 5. Separate parking lanes at the Leien of Antwerp with photocatalytic pavement blocks.

led to new trial applications in which people have tried to establish the relation between the results in the laboratory and the real effect on site, see e.g., [23–25]. In this section an overview is given of two such recent projects in Belgium which were implemented in collaboration with the BRRC.

5.5.1. LIFE+ PROJECT PHOTOPAQ

The European Life+ funded project PhotoPAQ [18] was aimed at demonstrating the usefulness of photocatalytic construction materials for air purification purposes in an urban environment. Eight partners from five different European countries participated in the project.

In this framework, an extensive three-step field campaign was organized in the Leopold II tunnel in Brussels, from June 2011 till January 2013 [26,27]. A photocatalytic cementitious coating material (TX Active® white Skim Coat from CTG Italcementi Group) was applied on the side walls and roof (total area of about 2700 m^2) of a tunnel section of about 160 m in length in one of the tunnel tubes directing to the city center. The air-purifying product was activated by a dedicated UV lighting system

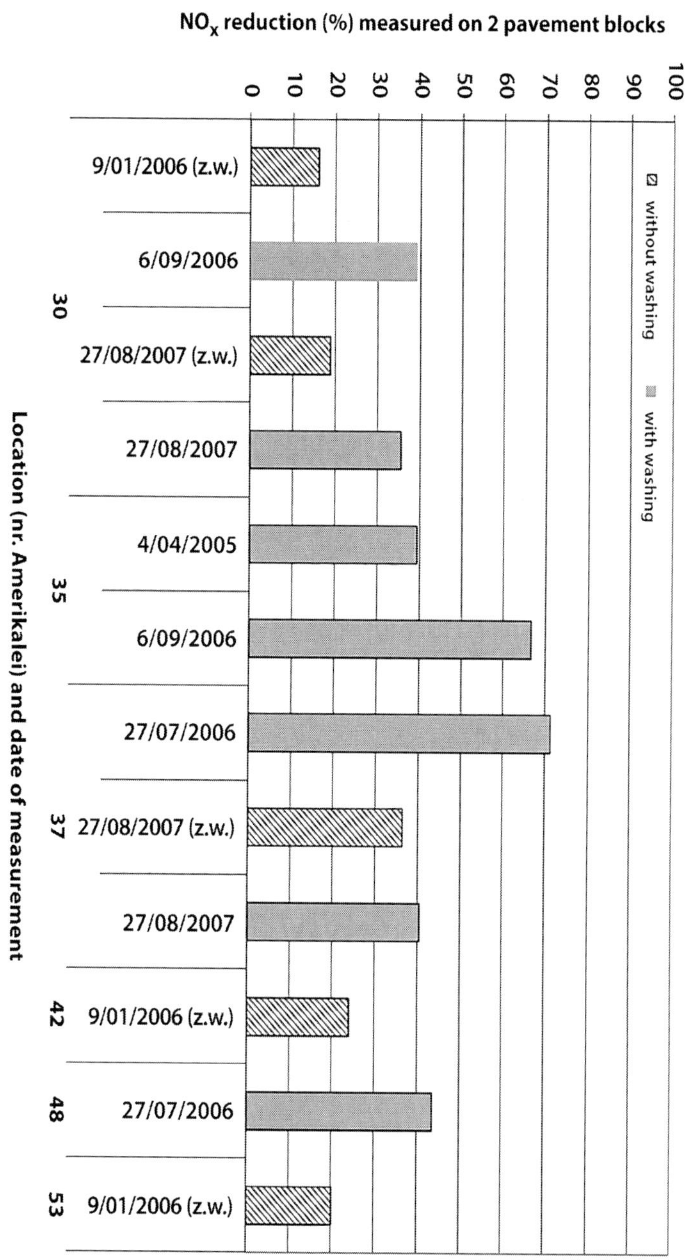

Figure 6. NO_x reduction measured on two pavement blocks, before (hatched) and after (colored) washing the surface, taken on different locations (house nr. 30, 35, 37, 42, 48, 53) and at different times at the Amerikalei in Antwerp.

(including Supratec "HTC 241 R7s" light bulbs from Osram, see Figure 7). More details can be found in [26,27].

Possible advantages of purifying the tunnel air may be, obviously, cleaner air to breathe, with a potentially reduced need of ventilation, but also (and maybe mainly) a reduction of the pollution impact of tunnel exhaust on the city air quality. During the field campaigns, the effect of the photocatalytic coating on the air pollution (including NO_x, VOC's, particulate matter, CO, etc.) inside the tunnel section was rigorously assessed.

The PhotoPAQ consortium mobilized a large panel of up-to-date instrumentations, installed in the tunnel for several weeks, aiming at characterizing the levels of pollution in this section of the Leopold II tunnel, with and without the air-purifying product (Figure 8).

However, in contrast to first estimations based on laboratory studies, the results indicated no observable reduction of the pollution level, i.e., the reduction of nitrogen oxides (NO_x, one of the major traffic related air pollutants) is below 2%, which is the experimental uncertainty of the measurements.

A severe de-activation of the photocatalytic material was observed inside the highly trafficked and strongly polluted Leopold II tunnel. In conjunction, final UV lighting intensity (only 2 W/m^2 UV-A) was below the targeted values (above 4 W/m^2), which led to too low levels for proper activation inside the polluted tunnel environment. Another negative condition was the high wind speed (up to 3 m/s) inside the tunnel, limiting the contact time between pollutants and the active surface. Finally, January 2013 turned out to be an unusually wintry period causing cold and humid conditions inside the tunnel, with relative humidity ranging from 70% to 90%, which also reduces the activity of the photocatalytic material as shown before. Thus, all these issues together resulted in a reduction of the activity of the photocatalytic surfaces inside the harsh environment of the Leopold II tunnel, by a factor of 10 compared to the theoretical expectations. More details about the set-up and results of these extensive field campaigns inside the Leopold II tunnel are presented elsewhere [26,27].

Nevertheless, combining the knowledge gained during these campaigns and the laboratory based investigations performed by the PhotoPAQ consortium, numerical simulations (with the commercially available general

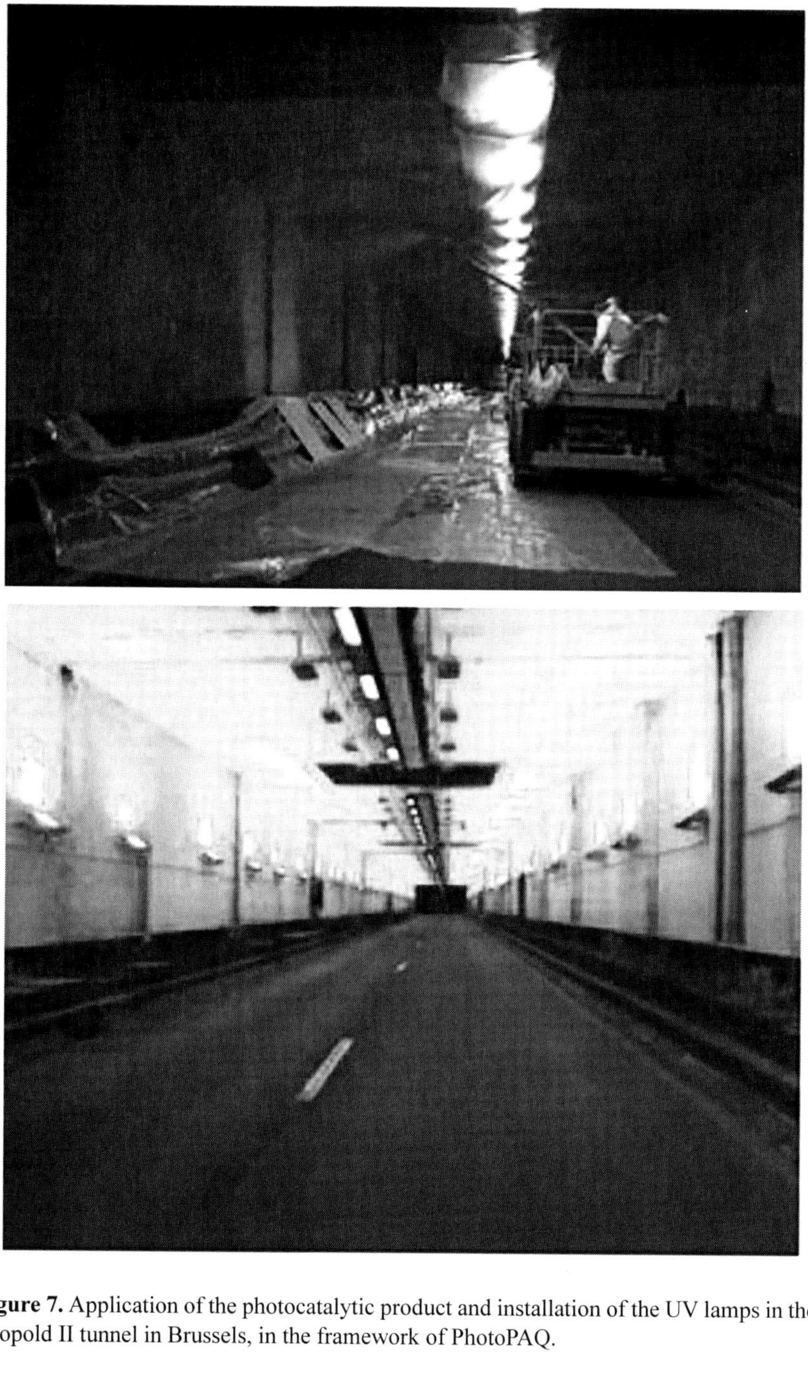

Figure 7. Application of the photocatalytic product and installation of the UV lamps in the Leopold II tunnel in Brussels, in the framework of PhotoPAQ.

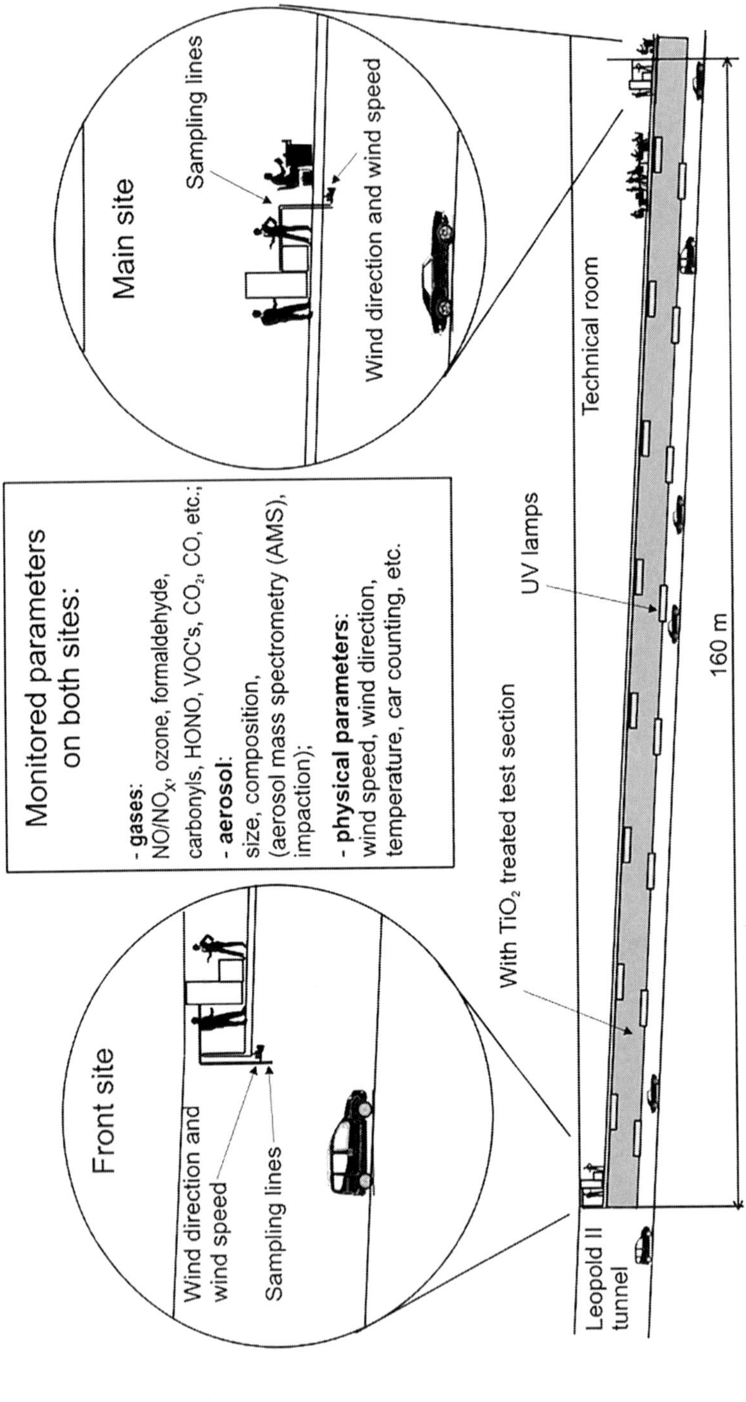

Figure 8. Full characterization of the air quality inside the tunnel test section during the PhotoPAQ campaigns.

purpose Computational Fluid Dynamics code ANSYS CFX®) were performed in order to estimate the possible best-case abatement of pollutants.

These calculations indicate that, under the best case scenario (proper level of UV light intensity higher than 4 W/m^2, relative humidity below 50%, and limited pollution to avoid passivation), the reduction of the NO_x concentration may be expected to attain:

- ±3% for the 160 m long test section;
- ±12% for the entire Leopold II tunnel (ca. 3 km), if not affected by ventilation.

Despite the fact that the results were not as expected, the Leopold II field campaigns conducted by the PhotoPAQ team proved to be a unique real world and fully comprehensive assessment of the effect of photocatalytic air-purifying (road) construction materials on air pollution inside a tunnel environment. Based on the extensive experimental data set gathered and numerical model calculations, a valuable tool for extrapolation can be provided to estimate the expected pollution reduction in other urban tunnel sites, also for use by non-experts [18].

5.5.2. INTERREG PROJECT ECO$_2$PROFIT

The broad environmental sustainability project ECO$_2$PROFIT dealt with the reduction of the emission of greenhouse gases and sustainable production of energy on industrial estates in the frontier area between Flanders and Holland. To reach these goals, several tangible demonstration projects were carried out on industrial sites in Belgium and the Netherlands. BRRC was involved in two such projects: "Den Hoek 3" in Wijnegem and "Duwijckpark" in Lier (both near Antwerp). Here, the regional development agency POM Antwerp was aiming to use a double layered concrete for the road construction, with recycled concrete aggregates in the bottom layer and photocatalytic materials (TiO_2) in the top layer, using photoactive cements and/or coatings. That way, air purifying and CO_2 reducing concrete roads could be built which are both innovating and energy efficient.

For these recently completed applications (2010–2011) BRRC was asked to set-up an elaborate testing program in the lab to help optimize the air purifying performance of the top layer, without interfering with other properties of the concrete (workability, strength, durability etc.). In the construction site of Wijnegem (Den Hoek 3), it was opted to use an exposed aggregates surface finish (with grain size between 0 and 6.3 mm) on the top layer for reasons of noise reduction and comfort of the road user. For the site in Lier (Duwijckpark) a brushed surface finishing was chosen to have more active cement at the surface. Indeed, the type of surface finishing and/or treatment of the pavement can have an effect on the photocatalytic efficiency, as shown in Figure 9 for three types of surface finishing: exposed aggregates, smooth (formwork side) and sawn surface. The results show that the exposed aggregates surface performs equally well as the smooth, formwork surface, but not as good as a sawn surface. This is the result of the combined action of less photoactive cement at the surface and a higher surface porosity (higher specific surface), two competing effects which in the end yield the final efficiency shown in Figure 9.

For the application of photocatalytic materials in a concrete road (and in general for any other type of application) a fundamental choice can be made between: mixing in the mass (e.g., TiO_2 in cement) and/or spraying on the surface (suspension of TiO_2). The former has the advantage of a more durable action since the TiO_2 will continuously be present, even after wearing of the top layer. On the other hand, the initial cost will be higher (higher TiO_2 content, necessity for double layered concrete) and only the TiO_2 at the surface will be active. In contrast, dispersing at the surface of a TiO_2 solution will provide a more direct action, and a lower initial cost (e.g., "ordinary" cement). In this case however, the longevity of the photocatalytic action could be questioned because of loss of adhesion to the surface in time. This fundamental choice was also investigated within the research program, together with the influence of several other parameters [28].

The effect of a curing compound for instance—generally applied to protect the young concrete against desiccation in Belgium and placed directly after concreting or after exposing the aggregates at the surface in case of denudation—is illustrated in Figure 10. From this, it appears the curing compound will initially inhibit the photocatalytic reaction, most likely because it is shielding off the "active" components from the pollutants in the air. Consequently, it is probable that the curing must disappear from the surface, i.e., under influence of traffic or weathering, before the TiO_2 will reach its optimal air purifying performance. In case of a photocatalytic spray coating, this also means that it is best to apply the TiO_2 dispersion some months after the curing compound to have the most durable effect. Alternatively, the exposed aggregates concrete can be covered with a plastic sheet to prevent dehydration (in case the concrete surface is denuded).

More detailed results of the laboratory research can be found in [28] and [29]. Based on the findings and the optimization of the concrete composition, a proper selection of photocatalytic materials and application techniques could be made, for the construction of double layered, photocatalytic concrete roads on the industrial zone "Den Hoek 3" in Wijnegem.

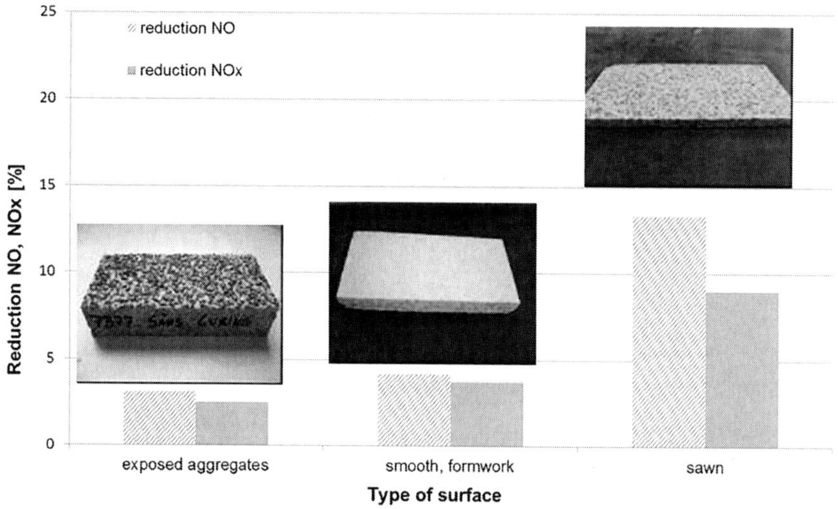

Figure 9. Effect of surface treatment on photocatalytic efficiency (only one type of "less" active product in mass).

5.5.2.1 DOUBLE LAYERED CONCRETE AT "DEN HOEK 3" IN WIJNEGEM

The concrete pavement of the industrial zone in Wijnegem has been constructed between the 15th and 18th of March 2011. The concrete was placed in two layers, wet-in-wet, with an interval time of approximately 1 hour. The bottom layer had a thickness of 180 mm, while the top layer was designed to be 50 mm. For the concrete of the bottom layer, 57% of the coarse aggregates were replaced by recycled concrete aggregates. For the top layer with TiO_2, commercially available white cement with 4% TiO_2 pre-mixed (by weight) was applied (CBR, Belgium, Heidelberg Cement Group). Two slip form pavers were used to place the concrete. As can be seen in Figure 11a, the color of the top layer is much lighter, due to the use of white cement and the presence of the TiO_2 (about 0.8 wt% of the top layer).

More information on the concrete composition, the execution and the results obtained in the lab as well as on site can be found in [28] and [29]. Besides the photocatalytic concrete roads, photocatalytic pavement blocks were also used for the bicycle lanes, parking spaces and foot paths.

Since this was a completely new industrial zone, it was not possible to have measurements on site before putting the photocatalytic concrete in place. An overview of the project is given in Figure 12. Immediately after concreting, a retarding agent was sprayed on the surface to be able to wash out the top surface after 24 h, to create an exposed aggregates surface finish (see Figure 11b). In order to prevent dehydration of the concrete during the first days, some parts of the road have been treated with curing compound; the other zones were covered with a plastic sheet. This way, the influence of the curing compound on the short and long term photocatalytic efficiency could be investigated.

The photocatalytic efficiency of the top layer was measured in two ways: in the laboratory on cores taken from the surface at the places indicated in Figure 12a, and "on site" with a special measuring set-up, shown in Figure 12b. This "on site" test is developed to evaluate the photocatalytic properties of the concrete pavement over time and to compare the different sites (with and without curing, for example). It does not measure the overall purification of the air around the pavement but enables to measure the durability of the photocatalytic efficiency.

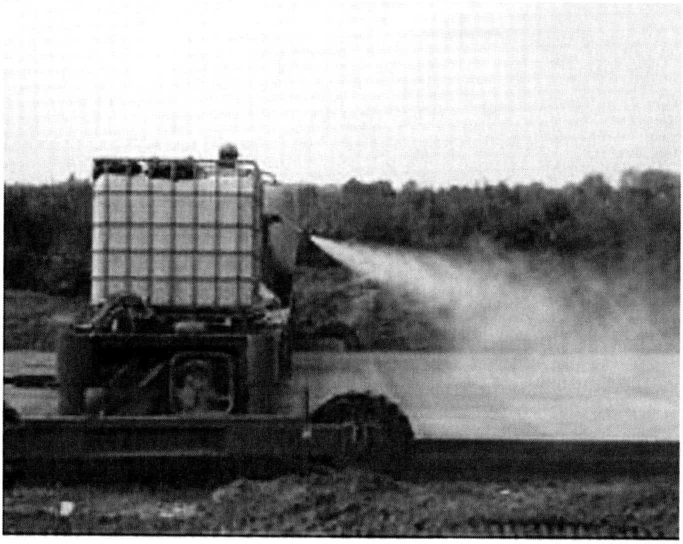

(a)

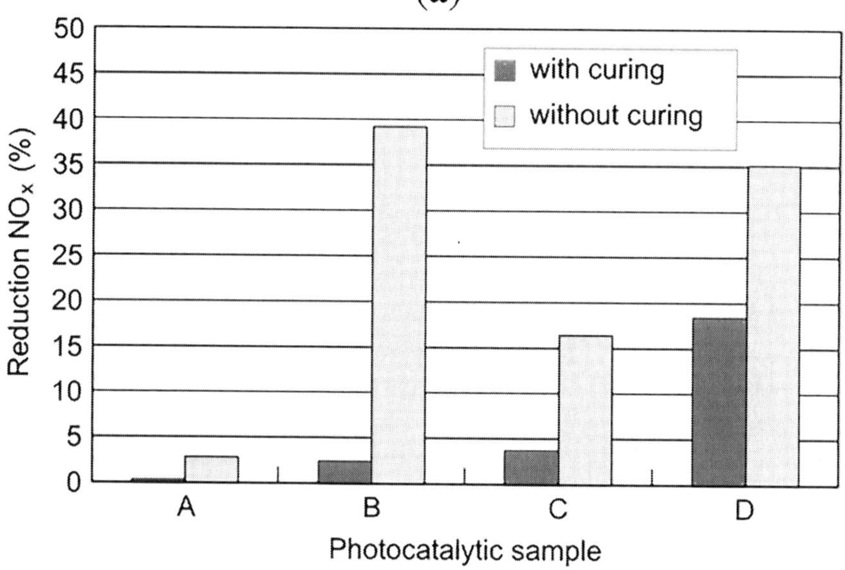

(b)

Figure 10. (a) Application of curing compound on fresh concrete, and (b) Effect of curing compound on photocatalytic efficiency (different samples A–D, with photocatalytic TiO_2 in mass and/or applied as dispersion, with and without curing compound).

The set-up consists of a Plexiglas frame, screwed air-tight on the test surface (concrete pavement), and is covered with a UV-transparent glass lid. The input NO-concentration (1 ppmv), relative humidity (50% RH) and air flow (3 L/min) are taken similar to the laboratory set-up. However, the total area covered by the box is somewhat larger (700 × 300 mm^2) to have a representative surface, and natural (varying!) sunlight is used in first instance to activate the surface. First results of the measurements o site are given in Figures 13 and 14, and were collected 5 months after the placement of the concrete (August 2011) at the places indicated in Figure 12a (points 1 and 2).

First of all, the results shown in Figures 13 and 14 indicate a large influence of the relative humidity (red curves). The NO_x abatement is lower when the relative humidity increases and higher when RH decreases again. The influence of the sun light intensity (measured through the UV intensity, light blue lines) is also visible, but on a different scale: variations over a shorter period of time do not influence the NO_x concentration immediately; it is the average sun light intensity over a longer period that is determining the attained NO_x abatement for the photocatalytic process.

Furthermore, the reduction in NO concentration is significantly lower for the zone with curing compound, indicating it is still (slightly) inhibiting the reaction: average reduction of 27% (with curing) versus 48% (without curing). Nevertheless, the effect of applying a curing compound on the fresh concrete (to protect against dehydration) seems to diminish over time. These results obtained on site (year 2011) are also in line with the results obtained in the laboratory, taking into account the difference in surface, relative humidity and light intensity [28].

In order to correctly compare the results between the lab and the field, the photocatalytic activity for NO_x (= sum of NO and NO_2) is expressed in terms of the photocatalytic deposition velocity in [m/h] under the assumption of a first order uptake kinetics and negligible transport limitations from the gas phase to the solid surface [30]:

$$k_R = \ln\left(\frac{c_o}{c_t}\right)\frac{F}{A}$$

where c_0 and c_t are the reactant concentration at the inlet and exit of the photo-reactor, respectively. In fact, this parameter refers to a first order

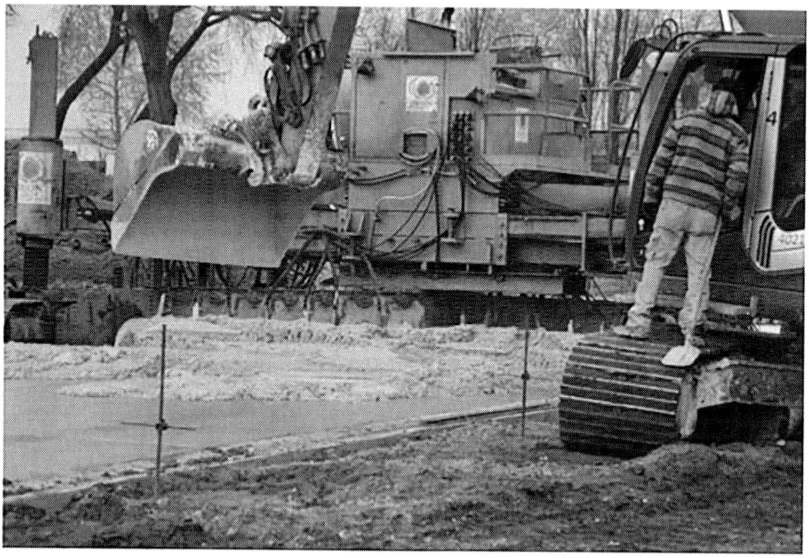

(a)

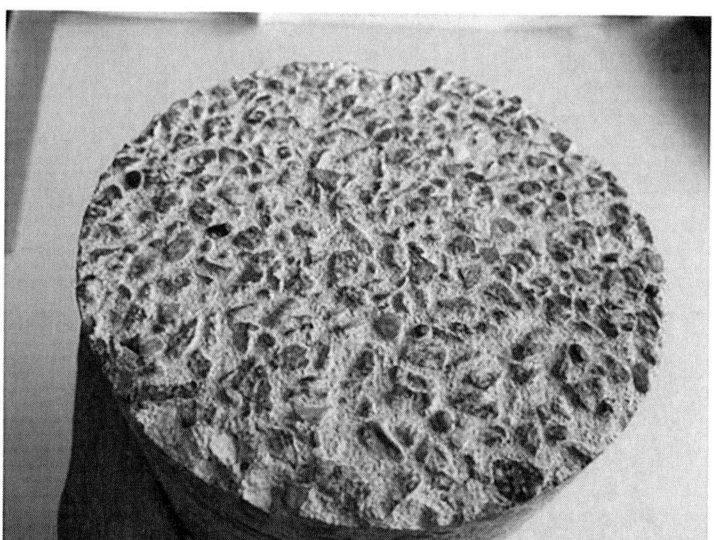

(b)

Figure 11. (a) Construction of double layered concrete pavement at industrial zone "Den Hoek 3" in Wijnegem; (b) Detail of exposed aggregates surface finish of the top layer.

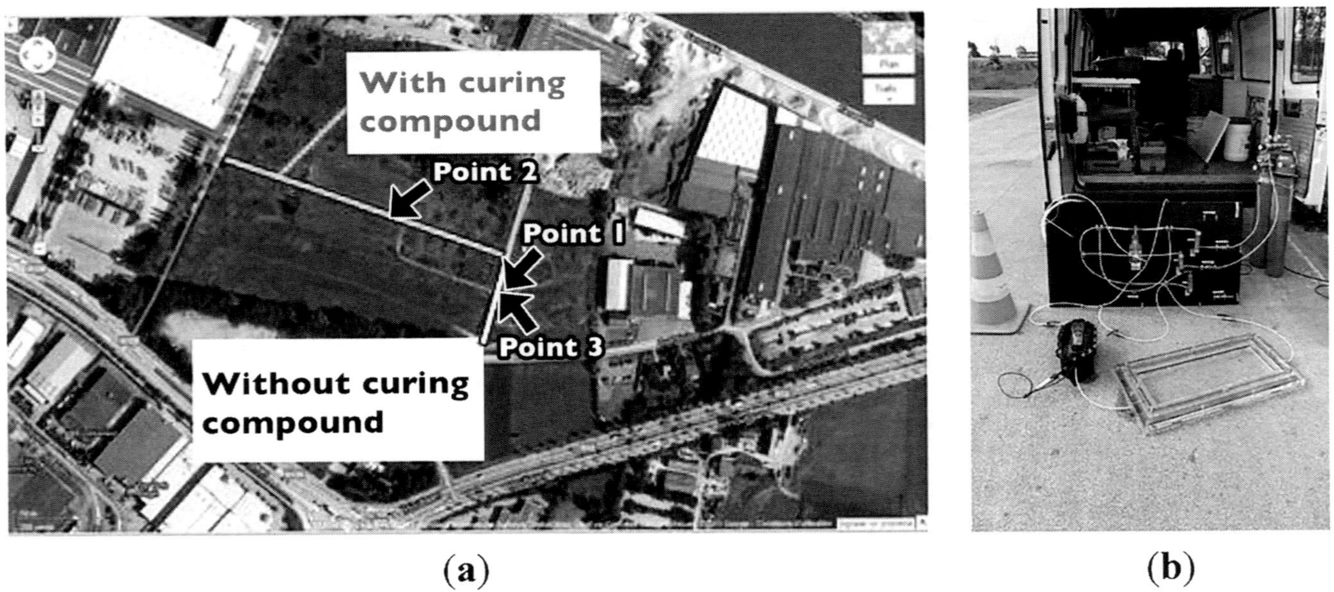

Figure 12. (a) Situation plan of the new industrial zone "Den Hoek 3" in Wijnegem, Belgium (Google Maps); (b) "On site" testing of photocatalytic efficiency.

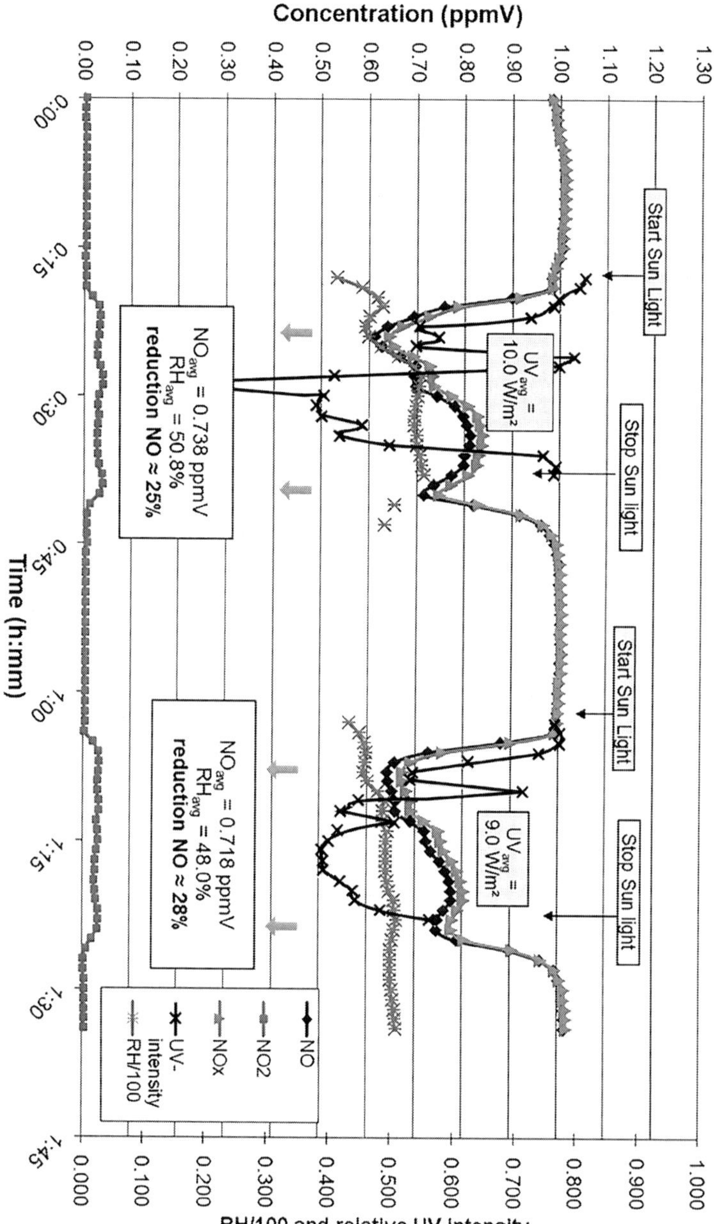

Figure 13. NO_x concentration measured at the outlet for zone with curing compound, 5 months after concreting (point 2, August 2011).

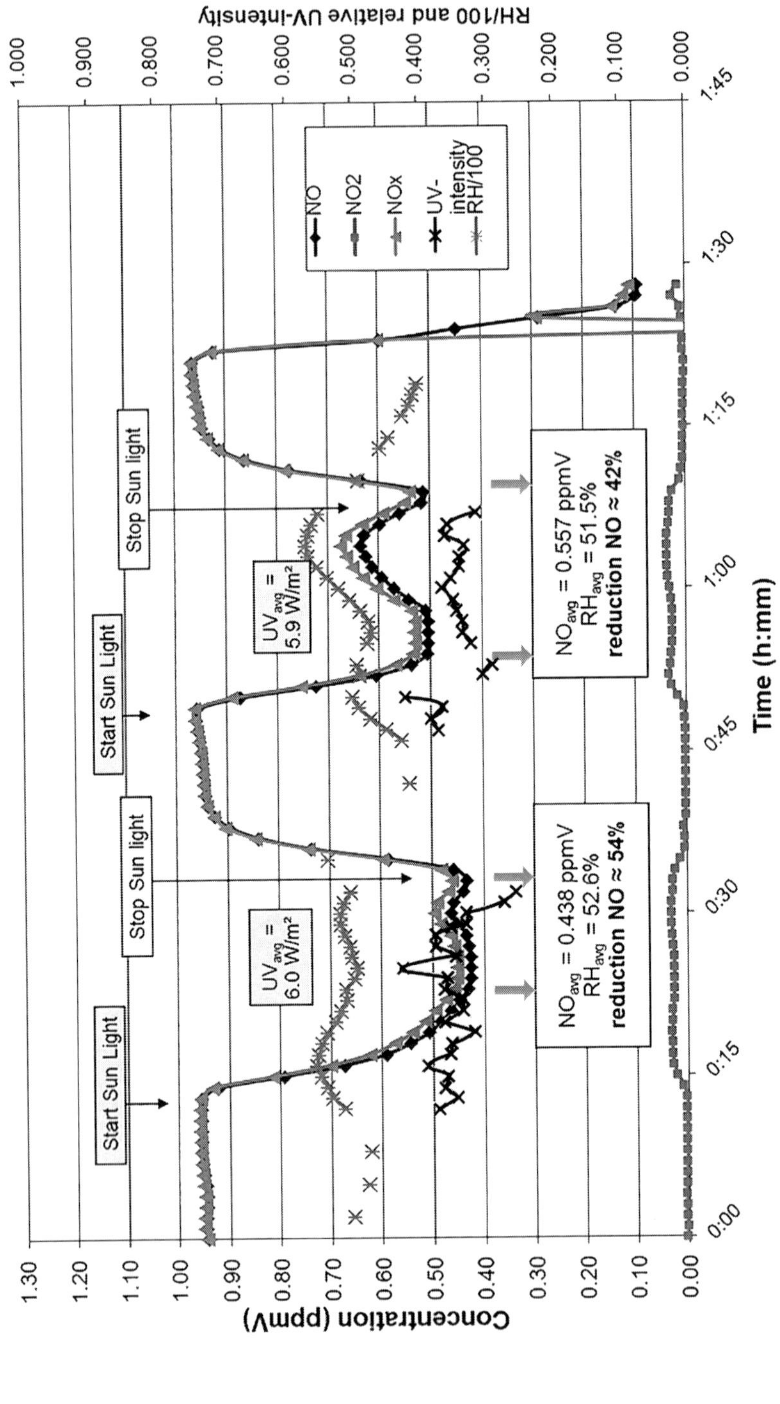

Figure 14. NO_x concentration measured at the outlet for zone without curing compound, 5 months after concreting (point 1, August 2011).

reaction rate coefficient independent of the applied flow rate F and the active surface (A) to volume ratio of the used reactor (lab or on site). In the lab work [28], average values for the NO_x deposition velocity $k_{R,NOx}$ of 0.25 and 0.70 m/h were obtained with and without curing compound respectively, which is in nice agreement with the results on site for 2011 (see further in Table 1).

The measurements on site are also repeated over time in order to see the influence of ageing and traffic on the photocatalytic efficiency. Recent measurements performed in the summer of 2012 for instance, are shown in Figure 15. Here, measurements were performed using an external UV-lamp (10 W/m^2) as well as natural sunlight to activate the photocatalyst present in the pavement. It appears the activity under sun light is somewhat higher compared to the UV lamp only. This could be due to the fact that the applied TiO_2 (in the active cement) is also partially active under visible light and/or is excited by the shorter UV wavelengths (UV-B, UV-C) present in the sun spectrum.

On the other hand, the measurement of the UV-intensity comprised in the sun light could be erroneous because of the radiometer used here. This is only calibrated for specific UV-A lamps (between 300 and 400 nm) applied in the geometry of the lab set-up which differs substantially from these exterior tests. The activity observed under natural, varying sun light though, is still very interesting from the view point of practical application. The use of the external UV-lamp with constant light intensity in turn, allows making a more absolute comparison of the photocatalytic activity between different zones and for different times.

In any case, the results of Figure 15 reveal already that the efficiency of this kind of photocatalytic application (TiO_2 integrated in the cement) appears to decrease in time: on average 34% NO-reduction (after 17 months) versus 48% (after 5 months). Possible causes could reside in the covering of the TiO_2 at the surface by dirt, the detachment of the TiO_2 from the surface or the deposition of products from chemical reactions which can take place at the surface.

In this respect, in October 2012 an aqueous TiO_2 dispersion (Eoxolit® consisting of a mixture of two different types of TiO_2 particles with a total concentration of 40 g/L TiO_2) was also applied on the surface in some parts of the roads on the industrial zone in Wijnegem, as shown in Figure

16a, for the purpose of comparative measurements. In total four different zones were considered:

- Zone 1 = double layered concrete (0/6.3 mm on top) without TiO_2;
- Zone 2 = single layered concrete (0/20 mm) without TiO_2;
- Zone 3 = double layered concrete with TiO_2 (active cement) and without curing compound;
- Zone 4 = double layered concrete with TiO_2 (active cement) and with curing compound.

The photocatalytic dispersion was applied with a dose of approximately 1 L per 5 m^2 on a total of 800 m^2, followed by spraying of a hydrophobic product for optimal functioning of the coating (manufacturers' guidelines). Important to mention however, is the fact that at the time of application there was a severe pollution with soil and dirt at the surface of the pavement in some zones due to the presence of a grinding installation plant at the site. This most certainly had an impact on the efficiency of the TiO_2 suspension (see further). Subsequently, provisional controls of the photocatalytic efficiency have been carried out to check the separate action of the two types of photoactive materials (mass and dispersion), and to further assess the durability of the air purifying performance. Most recent measurements on the site in Wijnegem were performed in the summer of 2013, at the measurement points (1–9) indicated in Figure 16b. All results obtained up till now (2011–2013) are summarized in Table 1.

First of all, when comparing the measurements on the surface of the pavement at points 1 and 3 (cf. Figure 16b) in 2013 with these of 2012, a very similar result can be noticed: a photocatalytic deposition velocity for NO_x of ca. 0.2 m/h under UV light. This indicates that the decreasing trend in photocatalytic activity for the concrete with "active" cement (see evolution 2011–2012) seems to be stabilized in 2013.

Furthermore, the measured efficiency for points 1 and 3 (in 2013) appears to differ little or nothing with the one for points 6 and 9, with application of the photocatalytic coating (TiO_2 dispersion) on the pavement surface. Here, the TiO_2 dispersion did not produce a significant added value (yet) in terms of photocatalytic air purifying action. Only for point 4 (active cement with curing compound, after application of TiO_2 disper-

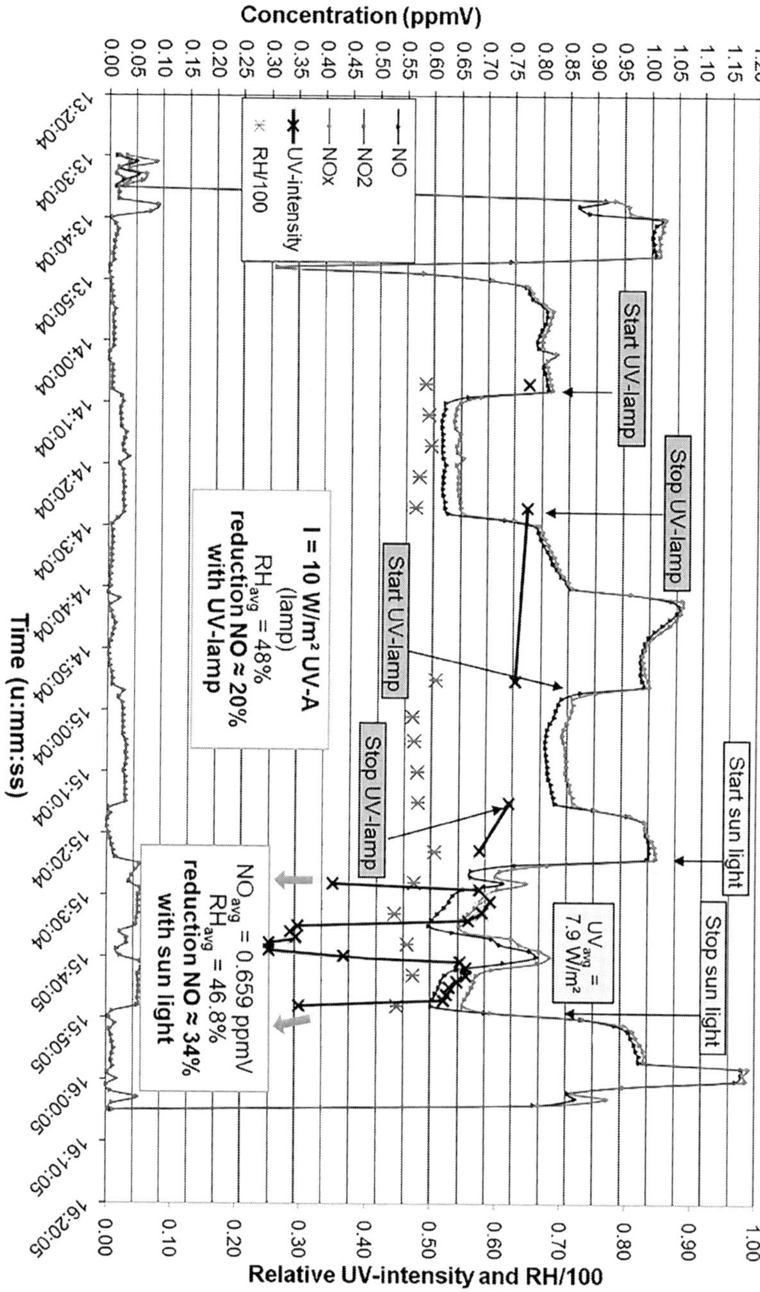

Figure 15. NO_x concentration measured at the outlet for zone without curing compound, 17 months after concreting (point 3, August 2012).

sion) one can notice a strong improvement of the photocatalytic efficiency (deposition velocity of ca. 0.8 m/h for NO under sun light and nearly 0.3 m/h under UV). Possibly, the pollution of the surface at the time of application has played an important part causing the adhesion of the coating to be far from optimal.

For points 7 and 8 (concrete without active cement, but with TiO_2 dispersion on the surface), the activity is not significantly better either (or even less) compared to the "pure" concrete with active cement. In addition, point 8 (single layered concrete 0/20) reveals much smaller photocatalytic reactivity than point 7 (double layered concrete with top layer 0/6.3): deposition velocity of 0.08 m/h versus 0.15 m/h for NO reduction under UV. This probably has to do with the stronger adhesion of the coating on the surface of the finer (0/6.3) double layered concrete compared to the coarser (0/20) single layered concrete.

Finally, a measurement on site was also performed for the newly constructed pavements at the industrial zone in Lier, which have a different surface finishing as illustrated in Figure 17a. The results of this measurement, 20 months after construction, are shown in Figure 17b.

In comparison with the measurements of Wijnegem in 2013 (see Table 1), a slightly lower photocatalytic reaction is observed in Lier, which among others is due to the use of a curing compound (for the brushed surface) and the lower TiO_2 content (less cement used). However, if we make the comparison with the zone with curing compound in Wijnegem (cf. point 4 in zone 4) measured in 2012 (17 months after construction), a significantly better result under UV light is obtained in Lier: deposition velocity for NO of 0.14 m/h in Lier versus 0.06 m/h in Wijnegem. This higher activity probably has to do with the brushed surface finish instead of exposing the aggregates (cf. Figure 9). In any case, these measurements confirm the photocatalytic action 20 months after construction of the concrete pavement.

5.6 CONCLUSIONS AND PERSPECTIVES

Photocatalytic (TiO_2 containing) paving materials with the potential of reducing air pollution by traffic are being used more frequently on site in

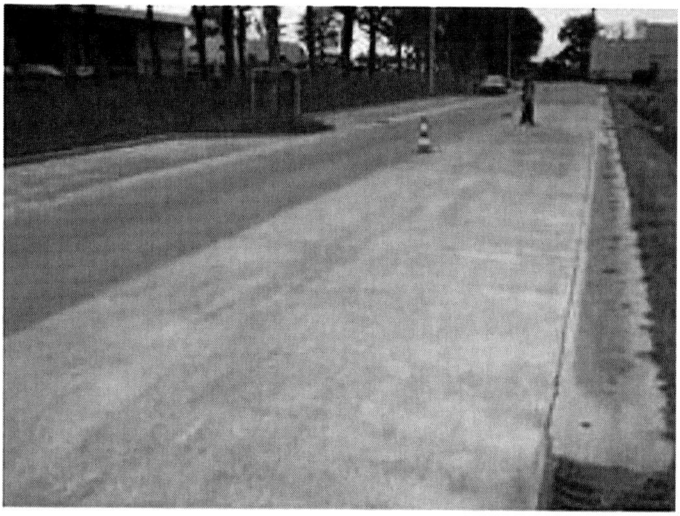

(a)

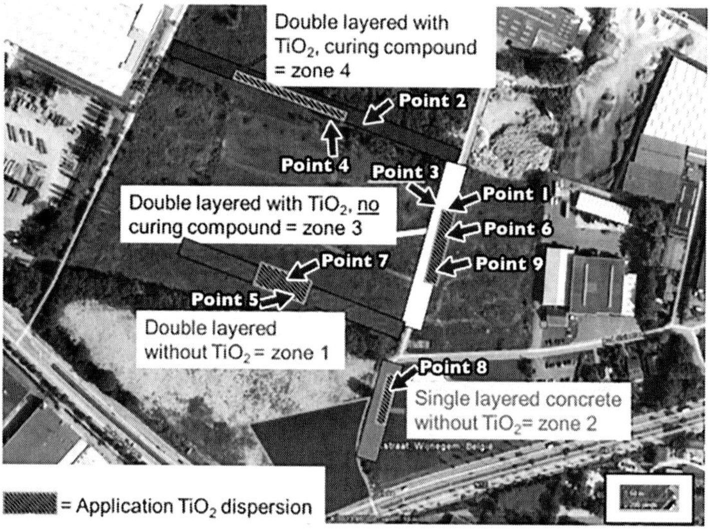

(b)

Figure 16. (a) Application of photocatalytic dispersion on part of the roads at industrial zone "Den Hoek 3" (October 2012); (b) Localization of measurement points for "on site" testing (Google Maps).

Table 1. Summary of results in time for photocatalytic activity measured on site in Wijnegem.

Zone	$k_{R,NO}(k_{R,NOx})$ [m/h]				
	Sun light			UV-lamp (10 W/m^2)	
	2011	2012	2013	2012	2013
4: with curing compound, active cement (point 2, 4)	0.30 (0.26)	0.09 (0.07)	-	0.06 (0.04)	-
3: without curing compound, active cement (point 1 and 3)	0.70 (0.66)	0.39 (0.34)	0.38 (0.28)	0.21 (0.19)	0.22 (0.18)
4: with curing, active cement +TiO_2 dispersion (point 4)			0.82 (0.62)	-	0.28 (0.22)
3: without curing, active cement +TiO_2 dispersion (points 6 and 9)			0.27 (0.20)	-	0.21 (0.15)
1: double layered, no active cement + TiO_2 dispersion (point 7)	-	-	0.32 (0.27)	-	0.15 (0.13)
2: single layered, no active cement + TiO_2 dispersion (point 8)	-	-	0.14 (0.13)	-	0.08 (0.07)

horizontal as well as in vertical applications, also in Belgium. Laboratory results indicate a good efficiency towards the abatement of NO_x in the air by using these innovative materials. The durability of the photocatalytic action also remains mostly intact, though regular cleaning (by rain) of the surface is necessary. The relative humidity (RH) is an important parameter, which may reduce the efficiency on site. If the RH is too high, the water will be adsorbed at the surface and prevent the reaction with the pollutants.

The translation from the laboratory results to the "on-site efficiency" is still a difficult and critical factor, because of the great number of parameters involved. Hence, there is still a need for large scale applications to demonstrate the effectiveness of photocatalytic materials in "real life" and evaluate the durability of the air purifying action, such as the European Life+ project PhotoPAQ and the industrial zones "Den Hoek 3" in Wijnegem en "Duwijckpark" in Lier. These recent applications in Belgium show already some interesting results.

It seems the use of photocatalytic cement-based coatings inside road tunnels is not mature for application on a large scale yet. From the experience gained during the Leopold II tunnel campaigns in Brussels, recommendations for the proper use of these innovative materials can be made though, such as:

- Optimized coating application for low surface roughness and minimizing dust adsorption;
- High UV light intensity levels in the order of magnitude of 10 W/m^2;
- Low average relative humidity of tunnel air ($\leq 60\%$);
- High enough photocatalytic activity, with threshold values defined from lab studies;
- Low average wind speed (< 2 m/s) in the tunnel for increased reaction time of pollutants;
- High surface to volume ratio (smaller sized tunnel tubes).

For the double layered photocatalytic concrete pavements using active cement, an efficiency comparable to the one measured in the laboratory is obtained initially; though it seems to decrease somewhat in time due to dirt build-up and other deposits on the surface, the air purifying action has

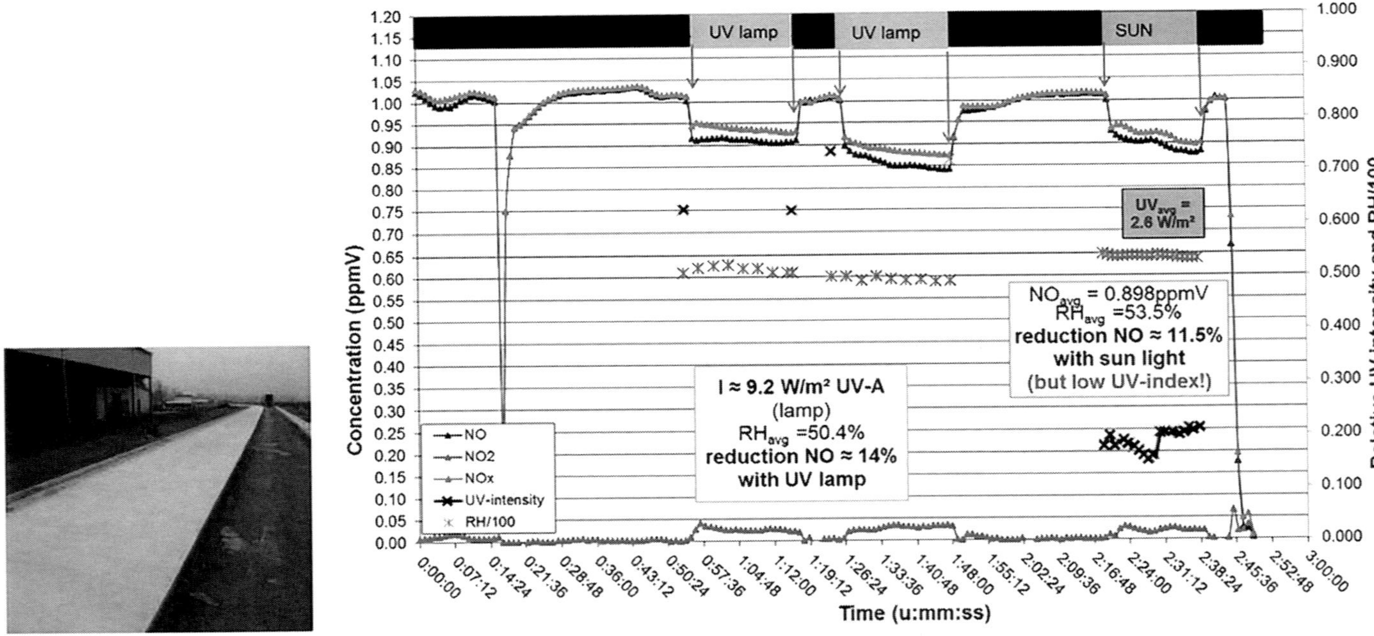

(a) (b)

Figure 17. (a) Double layered photocatalytic concrete pavement with brushed surface finish at industrial zone "Duwijckpark" in Lier; (b) NO_x concentration measured at the outlet for the site in Lier (active cement + curing compound), 20 months after concreting (August 2013).

stabilized after more than two years (2011–2013). Application of a curing compound—to protect the fresh concrete against desiccation—initially strongly reduces the photocatalytic activity and also has an impact on the long term. Use of a plastic sheet to protect the young concrete is therefore recommended. Furthermore, the exposed aggregates technique is not ideal for the photocatalytic efficiency since in this case a lot of aggregates are present at the surface and the TiO_2 is only present in the paste. The application of a brushed surface finish could lead to a better result.

Use of a photocatalytic coating (TiO_2 dispersion) on the surface of the concrete pavement does not produce an added value for the air purifying action compared to mixing in the mass, despite the good results in the laboratory. This probably has to do with the loss of adhesion in time and the filthiness of the surface at the time of application. Possibly, the coating is partially washed away with the dirt. In addition, better results are obtained on the finer, double layered concrete (0/6.3) than for the coarser, single layered concrete (0/20) which could be due to the better adhesion of the coating on the surface.

Durability of the photocatalytic action in time (for products mixed in the mass and/or applied on the surface) and optimization of the adhesion of photo-active coatings on the concrete surface, are topics that need to be investigated further.

Finally, the best results will be achieved by modeling the environment, validating the models by measurements on site, followed by an implementation of the different influencing parameters to assess the real life effect. One must bear in mind that photocatalytic applications are not effective everywhere; "good" contact between the airborne pollutants and the active surface is crucial and factors such as wind speed and direction, street configuration and pollution sources all play a very important role.

REFERENCES

1. European Commission. EU Energy and Transport in Figures, Statistical Pocketbook; Publications Office of the European Union: Brussels, Belgium, 2011.
2. Beeldens, A. Air purification by pavement blocks: Final results of the research at the BRRC. In Proceedings of Transport Research Arena—TRA 2008, Ljubljana, Slovenia, 21–24 April 2008.

3. Directive 2008/50/EC of the European Parliament and of the Council on ambient air quality and cleaner air for Europe. Off. J. Eur. Union 2008, L152:1–L152:44.
4. Chen, J.; Poon, C. Photocatalytic construction and building materials: From fundamentals to applications. Build. Environ.2009, 44, 1899–1906.
5. Renz, C. Lichtreaktionen der Oxyde des Titans, Cers und der Erdsäuren. Helv. Chim. Acta 1921, 4, 961–968.
6. Fujishima, A.; Honda K. Electrochemical photolysis of water at a semiconductor electrode. Nature 1972, 238, 37–38.
7. Fujishima, A.; Rao, T.N.; Tryk, D.A. Titanium dioxide photocatalysis. J. Photochem. Photobiol. C 2000, 1, 1–21.
8. Sopyan, I.; Watanabe, M.; Murasawa, S.; Hashimoto, K.; Fujishima, A. An efficient TiO_2 thin-film photocatalyst: Photocatalytic properties in gas-phase acetaldehyde degradation. J. Photochem. Photobiol. A 1996, 98, 79–86.
9. Cassar, L.; Pepe, C. Paving Tile Comprising an Hydraulic Binder and Photocatalyst Particles. EP-Patent 1600430 A1, 1997.
10. Murata, Y.; Tawara, H.; Obata, H.; Murata, K. NO_x-Cleaning Paving Block. EP-Patent 0786283 A1, 1996.
11. Ohama, Y.; Van Gemert, D. Application of Titanium Dioxide Photocatalysis to Construction Materials; Springer: Dordrecht, The Netherlands, 2011.
12. Saubere Luft Durch Pflastersteine Clean Air by Airclean®. Available online: http://www.ime.fraunhofer.de/content/dam/ime/de/documents/AOe/2009_2010_Saubere%20Luft %20durch%20Pflastersteine_s.pdf (accessed on 25 July 2014).
13. Dillert, R.; Stötzner, J.; Engel, A.; Bahnemann, D.W. Influence of inlet concentration and light intensity on the photocatalytic oxidation of nitrogen(II) oxide at the surface of Aeroxide® TiO_2 P25. J. Hazard. Mater. 2012, 211–212, 240–246.
14. Laufs, S.; Burgeth, G.; Duttlinger, W.; Kurtenbach, R.; Maban, M.; Thomas, C.; Wiesen, P.; Kleffmann, J. Conversion of nitrogen oxides on commercial photocatalytic dispersion paints. Atmos. Environ. 2010, 44, 2341–2349.
15. Devahasdin, S.; Fan, C.; Li, J.K.; Chen, D.H. TiO2 photocatalytic oxidation of nitric oxide: Transient behavior and reaction kinetics. J. Photochem. Photobiol. A 2003, 156, 161–170.
16. Ballari, M.M.; Yu, Q.L.; Brouwers, H.J.H. Experimental study of the NO and NO_2 degradation by photocatalytically active concrete. Catal. Today 2011, 161, 175–180.
17. Fujishima, A.; Zhang, X. Titanium dioxide photocatalysis: Present situation and future approaches. Comptes Rendus Chim. 2006, 9, 750–760.
18. PhotoPAQ (2010–2014) Life+ Project. Available online: http://photopaq.ircelyon.univ-lyon1.fr/ (accessed on 25 July 2014).
19. ISO 22197-1:2007 Fine Ceramics (Advanced Ceramics, Advanced Technical Ceramics)—Test Method for Air-Purification Performance of Semi Conducting Photocatalytic Materials—Part 1: Removal of Nitric Oxide; International Standards Organization (ISO): Geneva, Switzerland 2007.
20. CEN Technical Committee 386 "Photocatalysis" Business Plan—(internet) Draft BUSINESS PLAN CEN/TC386 PHOTOCATALYSIS. Available online: http://standards.cen.eu/BP/653744.pdf (accessed on 28 July 2014).
21. Hüsken, G.; Hunger, M.; Brouwers, H.J.H. Experimental study of photocatalytic concrete products for air purification. Build. Environ. 2009, 44, 2463–2474.

22. Beeldens, A.; Boonen, E. Photocatalytic applications in Belgium, purifying the air through the pavement. In Proceedings of the XXIVth World Road Conference, Mexico City, Mexico, 26–30 September 2011.
23. Maggos, Th.; Plassais, A.; Bartzis, J.G.; Vasilakos, Ch.; Moussiopoulos, N.; Bonafous, L. Photocatalytic degradation of NO_x in a pilot street canyon configuration using TiO2-mortar panels. Environ. Monit. Assess. 2008, 136, 35–44.
24. Gignoux, L.; Christory, J.P.; Petit, J.F. Concrete roadways and air quality—Assessment of trials in Vanves in the heart of the Paris region. In Proceedings of the 12th International Symposium on Concrete Roads, Sevilla, Spain, 13–15 October 2010.
25. Guerrini, G.L. Photocatalytic performances in a city tunnel in Rome: NOx monitoring results. Constr. Build. Mater. 2012, 27, 165–175.
26. Boonen, E.; Akylas, V.; Barmpas, F.; Boréave, A.; Bottalico, L.; Cazaunau, M.; Chen, H.; Daële, V.; De Marco, T.; Doussin, J.F.; et al. Photocatalytic de-pollution in the Leopold II tunnel in Brussels, Part I: Construction of the field site. Constr. Build. Mater. 2014, Submitted.
27. Gallus, M.; Akylas, V.; Barmpas, F.; Beeldens, A.; Boonen, E.; Boréave, A.; Bottalico, L.; Cazaunau, M.; Chen, H.; Daële, V.; et al. Photocatalytic de-pollution in the Leopold II tunnel in Brussels, Part II: NOx abatement results. Constr. Build. Mater. 2014, Submitted.
28. Boonen, E.; Beeldens, A. Photocatalytic roads: From lab testing to real scale applications. Eur. Transp. Res. Rev. 2013, 5, 79–89.
29. Beeldens, A.; Boonen, E. A double layered photocatalytic concrete pavement: A durable application with air-purifying properties. In Proceedings of 10th International Conference on Concrete Pavements (ICCP), Quebec, Canada, 8–12 July 2012.
30. Ifang, S.; Gallus, M.; Liedtke, S.; Kurtenbach, R.; Wiesen, P.; Kleffmann, J. Standardization methods for testing photo-catalytic air remediation materials: Problems and solution. Atmos. Environ. 2014, 91, 154–161.

PART III

MUNICIPAL SOLID WASTE ALTERNATIVES

CHAPTER 6

Case Study: Finding Better Solutions for Municipal Solid Waste Management in a Semi Local Authority in Sri Lanka

BANDUNEE CHAMPIKA LIYANAGE, RENUKA GURUSINGHE, SUNIL HERAT, AND MASAFUMI TATEDA

6.1 INTRODUCTION

A variety of studies on solid-waste management in developing countries have been conducted in recent years. Some researchers have looked at the influence of education to waste management [1]–[3], while others have investigated policy making for waste management in specific areas or countries [4]–[8]. Health and risk considerations around waste management have also been the focus of studies [9]–[12], while current systems of waste management in particular areas or countries have been analyzed [13]–[16]. Finally technology and engineering in waste management have discussed by some [17]–[19].

Solid-waste management, especially in developing countries, poses particular problems for each local community, so empirical field investigations are invariably required to solve particular local issues. Solid-waste management is emerging as a major problem for policy makers in developing countries as the quantity of solid waste generated has increased significantly and its characteristics have changed as a result of changes in peoples' lifestyles due to swift industrialization and urbanization. Rapid population growth and an increase in economic activities combined with a lack of education in modern solid-waste management practices, complicate efforts to improve the situation in these countries. Compared to high-income residents in developed countries, the urban residents of developing countries produce less solid waste per-capita. However, the capacity of developing countries to collect, process, dispose, or reuse the waste in a sustainable manner is highly limited. Recent studies have demonstrated the lack of capacity of local authorities to deal with this emerging issue and have recommended improvements at all levels of the administration systems to achieve a sustainable solution to the problem [4] [20] [21].

Several studies on waste management specifically related to Sri Lanka have been undertaken. Mallawarachchi and Karunasena (2012) discussed national policy enhancement on e-waste in Sri Lanka [22]. Solid-waste management conditions in Sri Lanka were reported by several researchers [20] [22]. A study conducted by Vidanaarachchi et al. (2006) especially showed that common causes of poor waste management in Sri Lanka are the lack of appropriate policies and legislation, lack of political and public commitment, and inadequate technical expertise at the local authorities [20]. Therefore, the development and implementation of appropriate policies, political will, and public commitment are essential in order to reduce environmental, social, and economic problems associated with the present disposal practices. In countries such as Sri Lanka, the problems associated with solid waste lie more with the present haphazard disposal practices than with the rate of generation. Therefore policies should be formulated to encourage solid-waste management practices through waste avoidance and reduction, re-use and recycling, and thereafter final disposal in an environmentally friendly manner.

The aim of this paper is to propose a solid-waste management program to eliminate the unsustainable waste- disposal methods practiced in a small local authority adjacent to Colombo, the capital city of Sri Lanka. The study focuses on identifying problems and finding solutions by conducting a questionnaire and pilot scale projects in the area, then proposing a municipal waste-management program that prioritizes waste reduction at source rather than recycling at end-of-life disposal. This study may also be relevant to similar local authorities in other developing countries.

6.2 BACKGROUND INFORMATION

6.2.1 COUNTRY PROFILE OF SRI LANKA

The Democratic Socialist Republic of Sri Lanka is located off the southeastern coast of India and covers an area of 65,610 km^2 between 5°55'N and 9°55'N and 79°41'E and 81°54'E. The Palk Strait separates Sri Lanka from India. Figure 1 shows a map of Sri Lanka with its nine provinces, three districts of western province (WP) and nine local authorities in Colombo District. Sri Lanka's population was approximately 20 million in 2012 with a per capita gross national product (GNP) of US$1395 and a growth rate of 7.7% [23].

6.2.2 LOCAL GOVERNMENT STRUCTURE

In 1987, Sri Lanka underwent decentralization of its government structure with the setting up of Provincial Councils responsible for carrying out activities planned by central government ministries and their departments and agencies. Currently there are nine Provincial Councils in Sri Lanka. The Provincial Councils comprise Municipal Councils (population of over 30,000), Urban Councils (population of between 10,000 and 30,000) and Divisional Councils (Pradeshiya Sabhas or Pradesha Sabhai) for smaller towns and rural areas. Currently there are 23 Municipal Councils, 41 Urban Councils, and 271 Divisional Councils. The Provincial Councils are responsible for supervising the functioning of these lower authorities, including their solid-waste management.

6.2.3 PRESENT SCENARIO OF SOLID-WASTE MANAGEMENT IN SRI LANKA

6.2.3.1 WASTE GENERATION

The quantity of municipal solid waste (MSW) generated in Sri Lanka has increased over the years with the growth of consumption patterns. Analysis of data has revealed that the amount of MSW per capita per day on average was 0.85 kg in Colombo Municipal Council, 0.75 kg in other Municipal Councils, 0.60 kg in Urban Councils, and 0.40 kg in Pradeshiya Sabhas. The primary sources of MSW are households and commercial establishments, while secondary sources are industries and hospitals. The major portion of the MSW stream in Sri Lanka is dominated by organic waste generated from households, markets, and slaughterhouses (Figure 2). The organic portion consists of banana stalks and logs, tree cuttings, sawdust, wood chips, and paddy husks excluding coconut shells. The organic waste is further grouped into long-term and short-term biodegradable. The former cannot be degraded easily within 2–3 months and is initially used as a bulking material in the composting process. The latter can be degraded within 1–2 months or even less. The moisture content and organic fraction of the MSW stream were significantly high with low calorific values.

6.2.3.2 RECYCLING PRACTICE

In Sri Lanka, waste separation at source is still not practiced on a large scale. Of the total MSW generated only 10%–40% is collected and the rest remains either piled up on the streets or dumped in low-lying areas, such as marshes and abandoned paddy fields. SWM practices in various local authority areas differ greatly. Although regular solid-waste collection systems exist in larger council areas, there is virtually no collection system in some of the smaller jurisdictions. The ratio of waste collected to waste generated ranges from approximately 93% in Colombo Municipal Council to as little as 5% in some of the smaller urban areas. In Sri Lanka, resource recovery from MSW has been developed informally over the past few

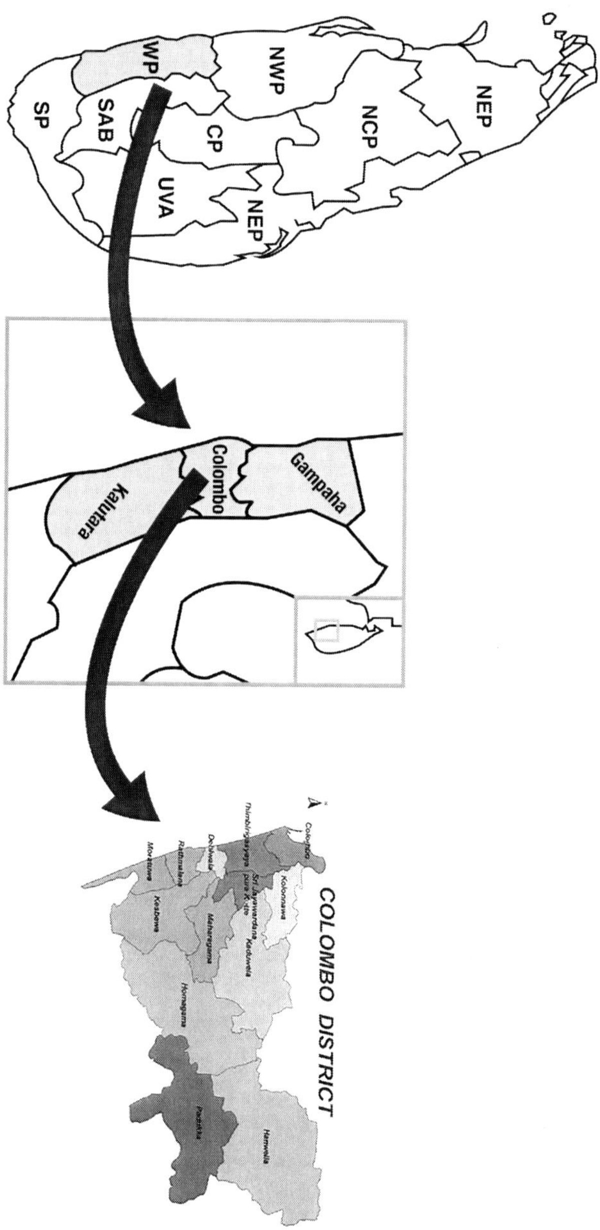

Figure 1. Map of Sri Lanka with provinces and selected districts and local authorities.

years for certain type of materials. Scavengers collect glass, paper, plastics, metals, etc. Currently, recycling of materials is carried out through an informal market system. Items are recovered at various points of the waste stream: at household level, during collection and transport by local authority workers, or at the final disposal site by waste pickers and municipal workers. The retrieved materials are sold to collection shops where they are cleaned and sold for recycling by local industrialists, or exported overseas. Also about 5% of the collected MSW is processed in various households and central composting systems. Household-level composting has proved more successful than centralized composting projects. The limited success of centralized composting is due to unsuitable locations and public protest against malodor and contamination of water bodies.

6.2.3.3 DISPOSAL PRACTICE

The most common method of final disposal of MSW is an open dumping, which accounts for more than 85% of the collected waste. These are non-engineered sites where waste is tipped haphazardly without environmental protection. The majority of open dumps are in the low-lying areas—marshes and abandoned paddy fields that are filled with solid waste primarily as a means of land reclamation. Some of the local authorities use a daily topsoil cover to reduce nuisance and allay public opposition. These dumps are used to dispose of every type of waste, including industrial, hospital and clinical, and slaughterhouse wastes, together with MSW, without any proper segregation. None of the open dump sites is engineered to manage the leachate or control pollutants released from waste decomposition. Few or no basic operations exist, such as leveling or covering of waste at the site, presumably due to the high costs involved. Soil cover is applied only at the final stage when there is a projected use of the land or public pressure. In addition to dumpsites operated by the relevant authorities, random dumping by private individuals takes place along streets, and on marshes and abandoned paddy fields. In the central part of the country, waste is mostly disposed of along the roads. Local authorities with regular responsibility take little control over these malpractices, mainly because ofa lack of resources or stringent laws.

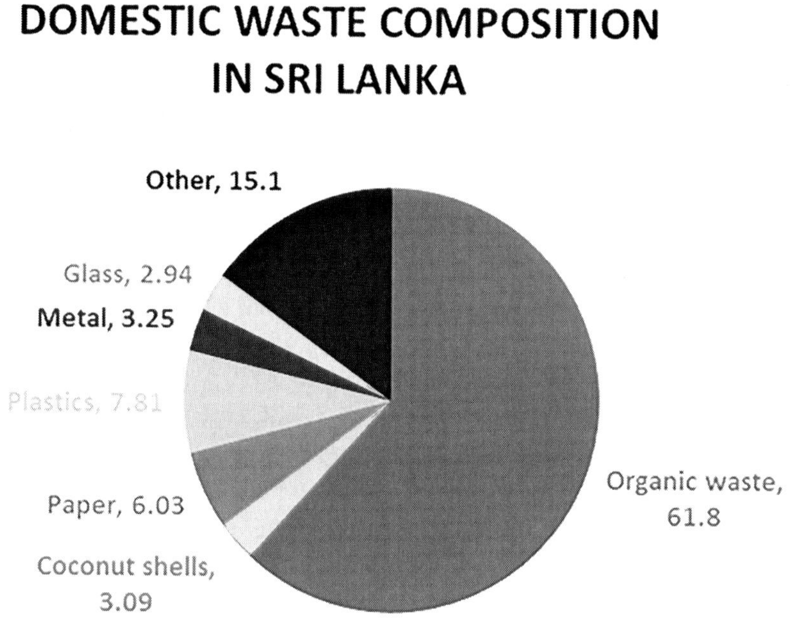

Figure 2. Domestic waste composition.

6.2.3.4 CURRENT PROBLEMS

Financial provisions for SWM in Sri Lanka generally fall under the health section of the annual budget of the local authority. The main source of revenue for local authorities is through property rates and taxes, supplemented by central government grants. There is no specification in the budget allotment for the various tasks involved in SWM. However, it has been estimated that local authorities spend around 3%–15% of their total budget on SWM. Practically all the local authorities spend more than 80% of the allotted budget in collection and transportation of refuse, of which a significant amount goes to salaries, allowances, wages, maintenance, and fuel costs. Most local authorities, with the exception of Municipal Councils and Urban Councils, spend hardly money on disposal, since the wastes are hastily dumped without spreading and compaction. The accumulation of uncollected MSW in public places and the improper handling of MSW during transportation, disposal, and scavenging have become major health and safety issues in Sri Lanka. Insects, rodents, and other vectors are attracted to the waste and can spread communicable diseases, such as cholera and dengue fever. Furthermore, use of water polluted by solid waste for bathing, cooking, irrigation, and drinking could expose individuals to diseases, pathogens, and other contaminants. Various diseases are spread via the fecal-oral route facilitated by unsafe water supplies and inadequate sanitary conditions. A lack of understanding of the causes of diseases related to garbage coupled with the existing bureaucratic approach to managing MSW, means the significance of health impacts and the potential threat to workers in the waste stream are often not recognized. For these reasons health aspects are often neglected by the government and the authorities.

Obstacles to implementing proper solid-waste management systems by local authorities in Sri Lanka include inadequate facilities for final disposal; introduction of improper solid waste management; lack of knowledge, technology and expertise about waste; poor planning and management; high cost of collection; and the attitude of people towards waste.

6.3 RESEARCH METHODS

6.3.1 STUDY AREA

The study area is in Kaduwela, Pradeshiya Sabha, which has a population of 252,041 (Department of Census and Statistics Sri Lanka, 2012) and is divided into three public health inspector divisions. The area is highly residential, having better infrastructure compared to the other parts of the country. The average daily waste generation is approximately 35 metric tons, which is gathered in a dumping area. The waste comprises both combustible and non-combustible materials generated from market stalls, households, and industrial sections. The dumped waste is then taken by Burns Environmental Technologies Ltd. (BETL), a private company. The Pradeshiya Sabha pays US$9 per metric ton to BETL and has to spend nearly US$10,000 per month on waste management. Despite this, large amounts of waste still go to the dumping area.

6.3.2 QUESTIONNAIRE

In order to obtain both qualitative and quantitative data, a questionnaire survey was conducted. The questionnaire was carried out with a random sample of 150 families totaling 750 residents from Battaramulla area, a major town in the Kaduwela Pradeshiya Sabha. The survey focused on the present MSW disposal practices of the residential community, their habits and attitude to solid waste, and the level of involvement of recycling, including home composting. The questionnaire method involved distributing questionnaires to representatives of each family and then organized a meeting of all respondents to collect the information individually. This resulted in a return of 100%.

6.3.3 FIELD OBSERVATIONS

Field observations were made on the quantity and composition of MSW in the same community that responded to the questionnaire. Initially the selected community was instructed to practice waste separation through an awareness program. The sorted waste was then transported weekly to the site and an analysis made for a month to determine the average daily values. The data obtained from this analysis comprised the composition of the waste, the quantities of waste available for recycling and incineration, and the moisture content. In addition, a detailed study of the waste collection system in Battaramulla town was completed.

6.3.4 PILOT SCALE PRACTICES

The proposed pilot project attempted to develop a better solid waste management system for a small local authority. The solid-waste management program for the treatment and disposal of waste suggested the following methods.

6.3.4.1 HOME COMPOSTING

Figure 3 shows the compost container selected for the project. The container was made of plastic and measured 1'6" × 1' × 6". It should not be exposed to rain. The total spending on the containers was about 2 US$. They had the advantage of being less bulky, portable, and providing quick composting performance, with compost being produced one month after installation. In households of six people about 2 kg of waste was put in the container per day. As this rate did not fill the container, this size would be suitable for one family.

6.3.4.2 INCINERATION

Given the category of waste available and the fact complete incineration was desired, a multiple chamber incinerator was selected [24]. The incinerator was designed with a waste feeding-rate of 289 kg/hr under a manual batch process. The size of the incinerator was 7' × 7' × 7' and the daily estimated operating time was 8 hours, using liquid petroleum gas (LPG) as fuel. The incinerator was designed for 15-year performance. The factor of increasing amounts of waste was managed by extending the operating hours of incineration. The temperature inside the secondary chamber was maintained at a level of 1000°C in order to destroy any unburned airborne particles. Installation of the incinerator cost approximately four million rupees.

6.4 RESULTS AND DISCUSSION

6.4.1 EVALUATION OF QUESTIONNAIRE SURVEY RESPONSES

Figure 4 shows the percentage of the community utilizing each disposal pattern of recyclable waste. Accordingly 38% practiced recycling mainly metal and glass by giving to scavengers, while 40% used the government waste-collection system. These results indicate that the public are not concerned with recycling at source, preferring instead to opt for the costly government collection and transporting system. Furthermore, 19% of the

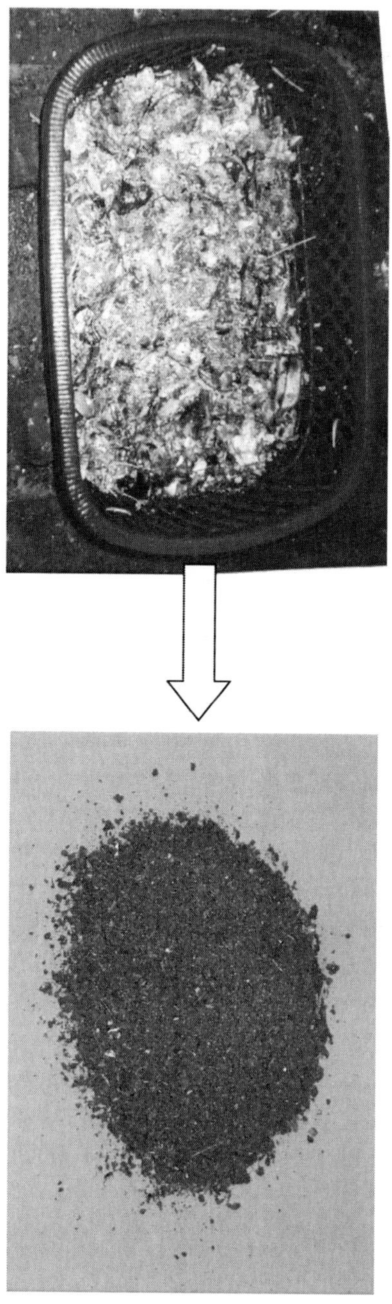

Figure 3. A composting bin.

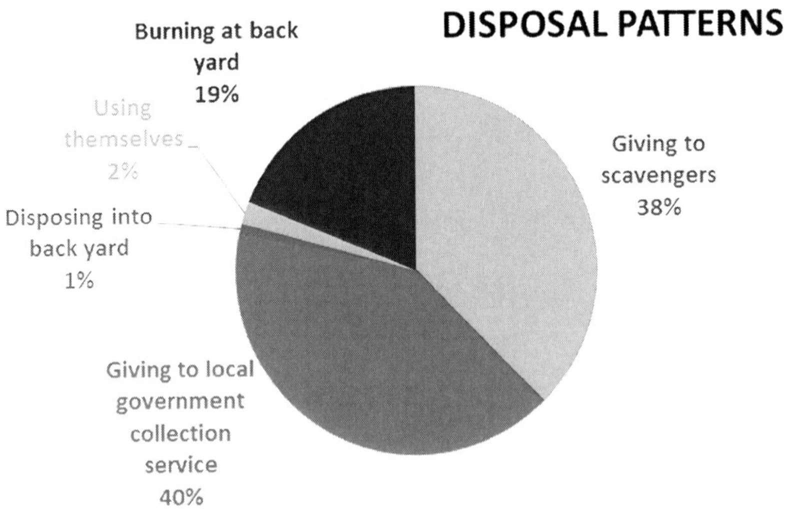

Figure 4. Disposal patterns.

community practice back-yard burning, which can be hazardous to human health because of harmful gas emissions, such as dioxins and furans, resulting from incomplete burning. This also shows that the general public is unaware of the dangers of such improper disposal methods. Figure 5 shows the percentage distribution of recyclable material collection. It indicates that people mainly recycle cardboard and coconut shells. They have not paid any attention to the recycling of other materials, indicating they are less enthusiastic about recycling. The questionnaire also revealed that the public consider the responsibility of waste disposal should be taken by the Pradeshiya Sabha and had a low awareness of solid-waste management, including waste reduction, reuse, and recycling. The survey also revealed that 40% of families in the community gave their organic waste to the government collection service, while 50% selected composting (data not shown). Of these, 97% preferred home composting using compost bins. They used low cost compost bins in preference to bulky bins.

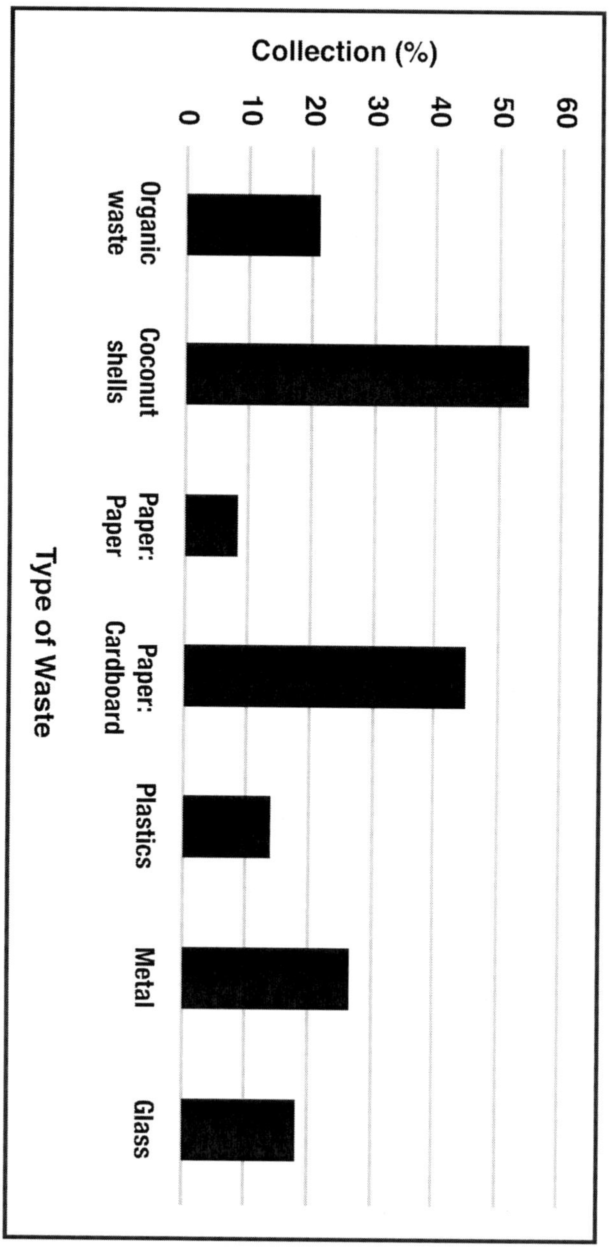

Figure 5. Collection percentage for recycling.

6.4.2 ANALYSIS OF FIELD OBSERVATIONS

According to Figure 2, as the major contributor of the waste stream was highly putrescible organic waste, it was important to promote home composting to divert this waste stream from entering the costly waste collection and disposal system. Accordingly, a suitable low cost compost bin was selected for this purpose. Battaramulla Pradeshiya Sabha collected domestic waste from supermarkets, garment factories, and hotels. Waste from Kaduwela and Battaramulla areas was transported and dumped at a one-acre site, which created health and environmental problems. About 35 tons of waste was gathered at the site per day. Before the disposal of such a large amount of waste, it is important to have a plan to reduce waste gathered at the site to simplify the process and avoid unnecessary spending. Therefore, attention should be given to reducing the waste. One way of doing this is to reduce waste at the beginning, that is, "at source". As domestic households are the main source of the waste, a "disposal at source" method should be applied. With this aim in mind, a solid-waste management program was carried out for a selected community as part of a pilot project and implemented to some extent by this project by applying proposed solid-waste management.

6.4.3 PILOT SCALE PRACTICES

Evaluation of the questionnaire on present disposal practices, along with the high organic composition of the waste, indicated that compost bins were a suitable method for disposal of the organic waste that had already been separated from other waste. The moisture content of the waste was about 65%—too high for the total waste to be suitable for incinerating, but composting was possible. Implementing such a management program in the whole Battaramulla area up to Kaduwela Pradeshiya Sabha would minimize the waste problem to some extent by virtue of the reduction of waste. The main problem is that the community did not want to buy the bins at such a high cost, although they liked home composting. Hence an experiment was carried out with a lower cost compost bin. This proved successful and compost was produced. With a low cost and easy handling, compost can be improved by trying better operation techniques. The total cost for the bin was only about 265 rupees and therefore affordable.

It is difficult to find a large enough land area in the Battaramulla region as the cost of real estate has increased. Considering the fact an incinerator is proposed as a suitable technique for the ultimate treatment method, it was also observed that 15% of the waste stream that cannot be reused or recycled contains materials suitable for combustion. Figure 6 shows the amount of combustible waste from 10 representatives from 150 families. Except for "Others" such as clothes/textile, rubber, leather, and so on, all types of waste were constantly generated in almost the same amounts from the first to the fourth weeks. As the total quantity of waste diverted for incineration is about two metric tons per day, an incinerator of less than one metric ton capacity was selected through literature review. The average moisture content of the waste available for incineration was 28%. Since waste for incineration should have a moisture content less than 30% the sample satisfied the scientific conditions. It was noted that the exhaust emission of incinerating certain waste, such as batteries, is harmful to the environment so it is recommended that further sorting of particularly hazardous waste be undertaken. Due to economic consid- erations, the feeding method may be manual using backhoes. There should be two or three laborers for the incinerator who can feed the waste manually with a capacity equal to the waste feeding rate. Although the installation cost of an incinerator is high, its operation could reduce environmental health problems expected from the improper management of putrescible solid waste, such as health disorders, sickness, and communicable diseases. The back-yard burning of waste causing air pollution could be banned as the combustible waste can now be sent to the incineration plant.

6.4.4 PROPOSED SOLID WASTE MANAGEMENT PROGRAM

The data analysis in this study indicates that creating awareness among the general public needs to be included in the solutions for the problems mentioned, as well as the provision of disposal methods, such as composting and incineration. Several studies, as listed in the introduction, have mentioned that education to raise awareness is necessary and important

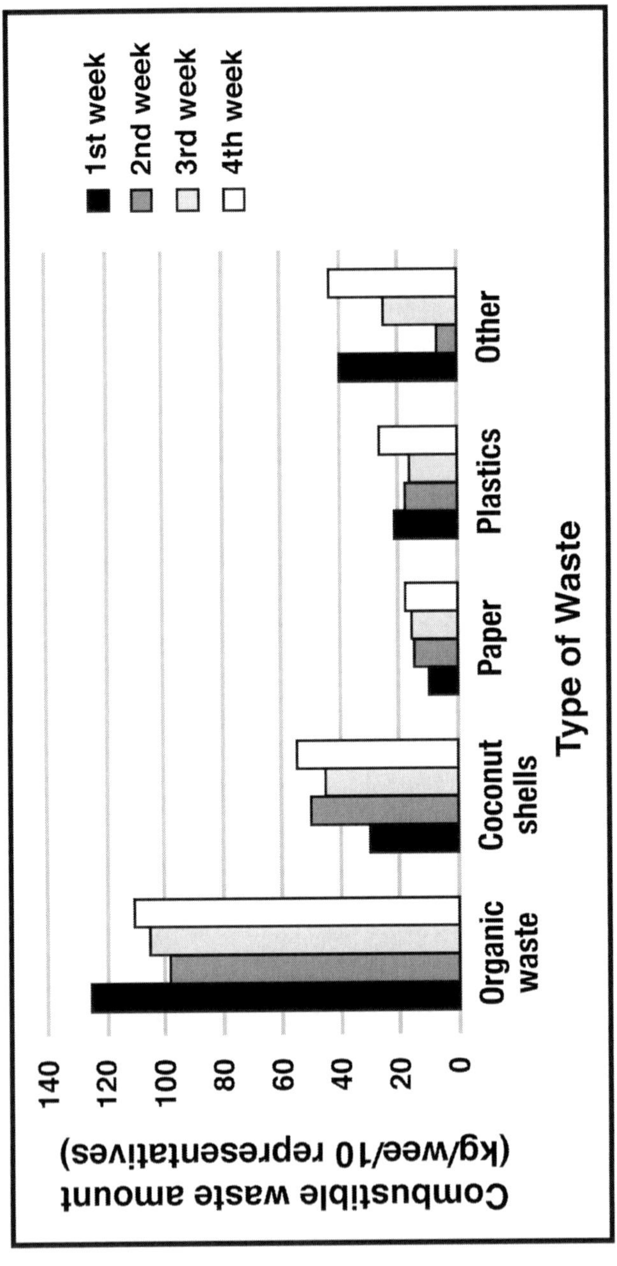

Figure 6. Combustible waste.

for waste management. Furthermore, the effective planning of solid-waste collection is important as this phase requires more than 75% of the total expenditure in SWM. In the proposed SWM program, special consideration was given to the separation of waste at source for the successful operation of the program. As the flow of some steps of the program depends on the feasibility of waste separation, final disposal methods are only provided for the separated waste stream. For the continuity of the program, follow-up is essential to ensure sustainability of the program and to avoid failure. Considering the above factors, the proposed so- lid waste management program is shown in Figure 7. An awareness program was carried out in the Battaramulla area based on a successfully implemented example of the community of Vijithapura, a good example society of the selected community. As a result of the implemented program the community has gained knowledge about waste avoidance, reduction, recycling, and waste separation. Also, after the awareness program was undertaken, sorted waste at source was mainly highly compostable—about 62.4%—indicating suitability for composting as a disposal method. Other recyclable wastes, such as glass, metal, and paper should also be given attention.

According to Table 1 income of about 5600 rupees per day can be achieved from recyclable waste. If the recycling project is carried out the 0.5 to 1 ton of waste sent to the site from the Battaramulla area could be reduced instead of being given to the BETL Company. However, a community-based recycling project could not be begun as the majority of the people are middle income and engaged in jobs with the public sector according to the information from the questionnaire and the interviews and the representative persons in the area.

After the community is educated to separate/sort the waste by the proposed solid-waste management program then it will be easy to collect recyclables, and scavengers can be referred to the sorted recyclable waste, as is being done at Vijithapura where these measures have already implemented, then the Pradeshiya Sabha can collect recyclables and obtain an income. However, theft of these recyclable wastes while being transported to the site has become a major problem. Another important factor that should be mentioned is that more than 5600 rupees can be earned by recyclables as long as they are not contaminated by waste. Out of the 35 tons taken to the site, about 11 tons (one third of the total

Table 1. Total income estimation.

Types of waste	Recyclable materials	Average amount (kg/day)	Money conversion rate into rupees (Rs/kg)	Total income per day (Rs/day)
Paper	Cardboard	287	6	1719
	Newspapers, magazines, etc	25	10	250
Plastics	Plastic mega-bottles	19	21	399
	Ice-cream containers, other food containers, cans	25	18	450
	Small bottles	28	1	28
	Poly sacks/bags	8	2	16
Metal	Ferrous metals	67	18	1206
	Other metals, such as aluminium	13	100	1300
	Copper	0.42	300	128
Glass	Bottles, grass cup cullet, light bulds, etc.	58	2	116
	Total	530		5612

waste) are from Battaramulla Pradeshiya Sabha per day. This can be reduced by two tons through incinerating, half a ton by recycling and 8.5 tons by composting. By these means, collection of waste to take to the site can be reduced. In the rolling out of the awareness program, the following should be well organized to gain the maximum participation of the community and prevent unnecessary (or double) effort, time, and expense: maximizing publicity, executing high-quality programs, minimizing the time that people have to spend on waste reduction processes,

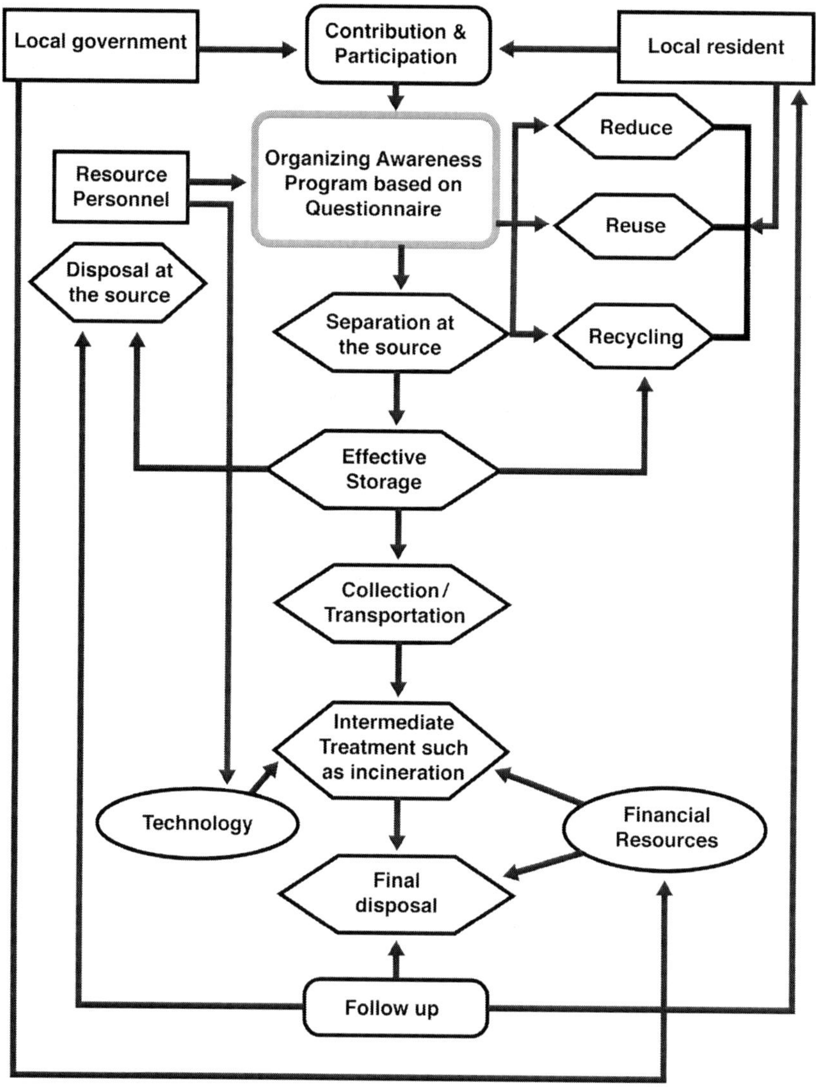

Figure 7. Proposed plan for solid waste management.

providing user-friendly leaflets and handouts, providing easy ways to participate, and gaining good information through questionnaires. Data from the questionnaire provided information on matters that should be considered in organizing awareness programs.

6.5 CONCLUSION

The study revealed that using solely engineering solutions for solid-waste management is not sufficient. As an example, collection and disposal of all the waste in the area are a complex and large-scale operation and require money to be spent on unnecessary storage, collection, and transportation. If the waste can be disposed of at the source, then waste can be eliminated at the point of generation and there then remains only a small amount for ultimate disposal. As the organic waste composition is high, the most suitable disposal method for the highly putrescible solid waste is composting. People are willing to use compost bins, and they require portable and low cost ones to do so. Hence to satisfy all the requirements, the proposed compost bin is suitable for the disposal of quickly biodegradable organic waste. Incineration is the most suitable method for the disposal of combustible waste. Although the installation cost of an incinerator is high, health and environmental problems will be reduced due to the complete breakdown of pathogens in the process. The bottom ash and fly ash, reduced to 5% of the input, can be used for land-filling, which is a benefit from incineration. If there is an option for alternative fuels instead of LPG, operating costs can be minimized. Awareness of solid-waste management is necessary and helps to reduce the waste problem in the Battaramulla area.

REFERENCES

1. Desa, A., Kadir, N.B.A. and Yusooff, F. (2012) Waste Education and Awareness Strategy: Towards Solid Waste Management (SWM) Program at UKM. Procedia-Social and Behavioral Sciences, 59, 47-50. http://dx.doi.org/10.1016/j.sbspro.2012.09.244
2. Jibril, J.D., Sipan, I.B., Sappi, M., Shika, S.A., Isa, M. and Abdullah, S. (2012) 3R's Critical Success Factors in Solid Waste Management System for Higher Educational

Institutions. Procedia-Social and Behavioral Sciences, 65, 626-631. http://dx.doi.org/10.1016/j.sbspro.2012.11.175
3. Sekito, T., Prayogo, T.B., Dote, T., Yoshitake, T. and Bagus, I. (2013) Influence of a Community-Based Waste Management System on People's Behavior and Waste Reduction. Resource, Conservation, and Recycling, 72, 84-90. http://dx.doi.org/10.1016/j.resconrec.2013.01.001
4. Rushbrook, P.E. and Finnecy, E.E. (1988) Planning for Future Waste Management Operations in Developing Countries. Waste Management & Research, 6, 1-21. http://dx.doi.org/10.1177/0734242X8800600101
5. Al-Khatib, I.A., Monou, M., Zahra, A.S.F.A., Shaheen, H.Q. and Kassinos, D. (2010) Solid Waste Characterization, Quantification and Management Practices in Developing Countries. A Case Study: Nablus District-Palestine. Journal of Environmental Management, 91, 1131-1138. http://dx.doi.org/10.1016/j.jenvman.2010.01.003
6. Zurbrügg, C., Gfrefer, M., Ashadi, H., Brenner, W. and Küpper, D. (2012) Determinants of Sustainability in Solid Waste Management—The Gianyar Waste Recovery Project in Indonesia. Waste Management, 32, 2126-2133. http://dx.doi.org/10.1016/j.wasman.2012.01.011
7. Menikpura, S.N.M., Sang-Arun, J. and Bengtsson, M. (2013) Integrates Solid Waste Management: an Approach for Enhancing Climate Co-Benefits through Resource Recovery. Journal of Cleaner Production, 58, 34-42. http://dx.doi.org/10.1016/j.jclepro.2013.03.012
8. Lohri, C.R., Camenzind, E.J. and Zurbrügg, C. (2014) Financial Sustainability in Municipal Solid Waste Management —Costs and Revenues in Bahir Dar, Ethiopia. Waste Management, 34, 542-552. http://dx.doi.org/10.1016/j.wasman.2013.10.014
9. Arukwe, A., Eggen, T. and Möder, M. (2012) Solid Waste Deposits as a Significant Sources of Contaminants of Emerging Concern to the Aquatic and Terrestrial Environments—A Developing Country Case Study from Owerri, Nigeria. Science of the Total Environment, 438, 94-102. http://dx.doi.org/10.1016/j.scitotenv.2012.08.039
10. Bleck, D. and Wettberg, W. (2012) Waste Collection in Developing Countries—Tackling Occupational Safety and Health Hazards at Their Source. Waste Management, 32, 2009-2017. http://dx.doi.org/10.1016/j.wasman.2012.03.025
11. Marshall, R.E. and Farahbakhsh, K. (2013) Systems Approaches to Integrated Solid Waste Management in Developing Countries. Waste Management, 33, 988-1003. http://dx.doi.org/10.1016/j.wasman.2012.12.023
12. Sasaki, S., Araki, T., Tambunan, A.H. and Prasadja, H. (2014) Household Income, Living and Working Conditions of Dumpsite Waste Pickers in Bantar Gebang: Toward Integrated Waste Management in Indonesia. Resource, Conservation, and Recycling, 89, 11-21. http://dx.doi.org/10.1016/j.resconrec.2014.05.006
13. Wilson, D.C., Velis, C. and Cheeseman, C. (2006) Role of Informal Sector Recycling in Waste Management in Developing Countries. Habitat International, 30, 797-808. http://dx.doi.org/10.1016/j.habitatint.2005.09.005
14. Oguntoyinbo, O.O. (2012) Informal Waste Management System in Nigeria and Barriers to an Inclusive Modern Waste Management System: A Review. Public Health, 126, 441-447. http://dx.doi.org/10.1016/j.puhe.2012.01.030
15. Paul, J.G., Arce-Jaque, J., Ravena, N. and Villamor, S.P. (2012) Integration of the Informal Sector into Municipal Solid Waste Management in the Philippines—What

Does It Need? Waste Management, 32, 2018-2028. http://dx.doi.org/10.1016/j.wasman.2012.05.026

16. Oteng-Ababio, M., Arguello, J.E.M. and Gabbay, O. (2013) Solid Waste Management in African Cities: Sorting the Facts from the Fads in Accra, Ghana. Habitat International, 39, 96-104. http://dx.doi.org/10.1016/j.habitatint.2012.10.010
17. Ouano, E.A.R. (1988) Review of the Issues in Hazardous and Toxic Waste Management in Developing Countries. Waste Pollution Control in Asia, 433-439.
18. Vehlow, J. (1998) Waste Management Systems in Industrialized and Developing Countries—Generation, Quality, and Disposal. Proceeding of First International Conference on Environmental Engineering and Renewable Energy, Mongolia, 7-10 September 1998, 405-414. http://dx.doi.org/10.1016/B978-0-08-043006-5.50057-4
19. Oakley, S.M. and Jimenez, R. (2012) Sustainable Sanitary Landfills for Neglected Small Cities in Developing Countries: The Semi-Mechanized Trench Method from Villanueva, Honduras. Waste Management, 32, 2535-2551. http://dx.doi.org/10.1016/j.wasman.2012.07.030
20. Vidanaarachchi, C.K., Yuen, S.T.S. and Pilapitiya, S. (2006) Municipal Solid Waste in the Southern Province of Sri Lanka: Problems, Issues and Challenges. Waste Management, 26, 920-930. http://dx.doi.org/10.1016/j.wasman.2005.09.013
21. Damghani, A.M., Savarypour, G., Zand, E. and Deihimfard, R. (2008) Municipal Solid Waste Management in Tehran: Current Practices, Opportunities and Challenges. Waste Management, 28, 929-934. http://dx.doi.org/10.1016/j.wasman.2007.06.010
22. Mallawarachchi, H. and Karunasena, G. (2012) Electronic and Electrical Waste Management in Sri Lanka: Suggestions for National Policy Enhancements. Resource, Conservation, and Recycling, 68, 44-53. http://dx.doi.org/10.1016/j.resconrec.2012.08.003
23. Department of Census and Statistics (2012) Census of Population and Housing in 2012. DCS, Colombo.
24. Bruner, C.R. (1998) Design of Incinerator System. McGraw Hill, New York.

CHAPTER 7

Incineration of Pre-Treated Municipal Solid Waste (MSW) for Energy Co-Generation in a Non-Densely Populated Area

ETTORE TRULLI, VINCENZO TORRETTA, MASSIMO RABONI, AND SALVATORE MASI

7.1 INTRODUCTION

The main objective in integrated solid waste management (ISWM) [1,2] is to implement technologies that reduce the environmental pressure by recovering both the fractions with a considerable value on the market and the non-traditional ones (e.g., organic [3–8], medical [9–11], automotive shredder residues [12], WEEE [13]). Moreover, any good management system also includes the involvement of the people, who have to be aware of the environmental benefits and of the reduced danger to health that results from a correct behavior [14,15]. Such an objective is highlighted by European Union (EU) legislation, which produced several Directives on waste disposal, treatment and incineration [16–19]. Such Directives: (i) prohibit waste recovery and disposal that have a negative impact on both the human health and the environment; (ii) aim at the reduction of waste production as well as the promotion of the reuse, the recycling and the recovery activities. The Italian Government acknowledged these Directives [20,21], also imposing the energy recovery from waste incineration.

According to the above-mentioned regulations and principles, the ISWM should both reduce landfilling and increase energy and materials recovery in order to lower environmental impact, energy resources consumption and economic costs. For example, landfilling of energy-rich waste should be avoided as far as possible, partly because of the negative environmental impacts of the technique, but mainly because of the low resources recovery [22].

Various types of Life-Cycle-Analysis (LCA) have been proposed for determining the most environmental-sound ISWM procedure [23,24]. Most of them focus on high percentages of separated collection in relatively small and densely populated area: some examples are described in [25–28]. However, in a scarcely-populated area, the environmental (e.g., GHG emissions) and economic impact of MSW collection is high because of fuel consumption [25,29,30]. The ISWM issue in a non-densely populated area concerns developing and developed countries. For example, 60% of EU surface has a population density of less than 100 inhab km^{-2} [31].

In order to reduce the landfill volumes as well as to close the MSW cycle, a solution can be the waste incineration with energy recovery [32]. Therefore, excluding direct landfilling of MSW, the solutions for ISWM are essentially three (Figure 1): direct burning of the raw MSW; accelerated stabilization of the whole MSW prior to incineration; MSW mechanical pre-treatment with secondary fuel (or RDF) production prior to incineration and organic matter aerobic stabilization (the so-called biostabilization) before landfilling.

Regarding the last solution, the mechanical pre-treatment of waste by sieving has aroused great interest, because it influences the MSW volumes addressed for both incineration and landfilling [33]; as consequence, the process reduces the environmental impact of the whole ISWM system. Sieving is carried out on raw waste and it allows separating out a flow of material that is characterized by a higher energy content (heating value,

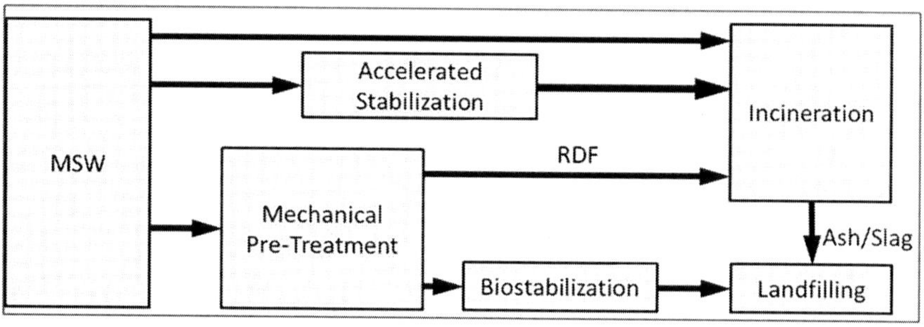

Figure 1. Typical municipal solid waste (MSW) treatment options.

HV, and net calorific value, NCV) [34]. The separation leads to a reduction in the combustion section, even if it partly penalizes the energy recovery. Moreover, in plants which treat waste coming from basins with different waste management policies, the pre-treatment process allows to guarantee a better quality of secondary fuel.

The case study presented in this paper regards the methodological approach applied to determine which technical solution may be proposed for solving some ISWM issues in a non-densely populated area, with specific reference to Basilicata, an Italian region. The analysis of the MSW composition and quantity (current situation and future trend) has been carried out. The results, combined with the waste size characterization, allowed to define the optimal mechanical pre-treatment in order to achieve an optimal balance between GHGs emissions and heat-and-power production.

7.2 MATERIALS AND METHODS

7.2.1 INVESTIGATED AREA

Basilicata is a predominantly mountainous region (Figure 2a) that covers about 10,000 km^2 in the center of Southern Italy. The population is less than 580,000 inhabitants [35]. Most of the 131 districts have a population

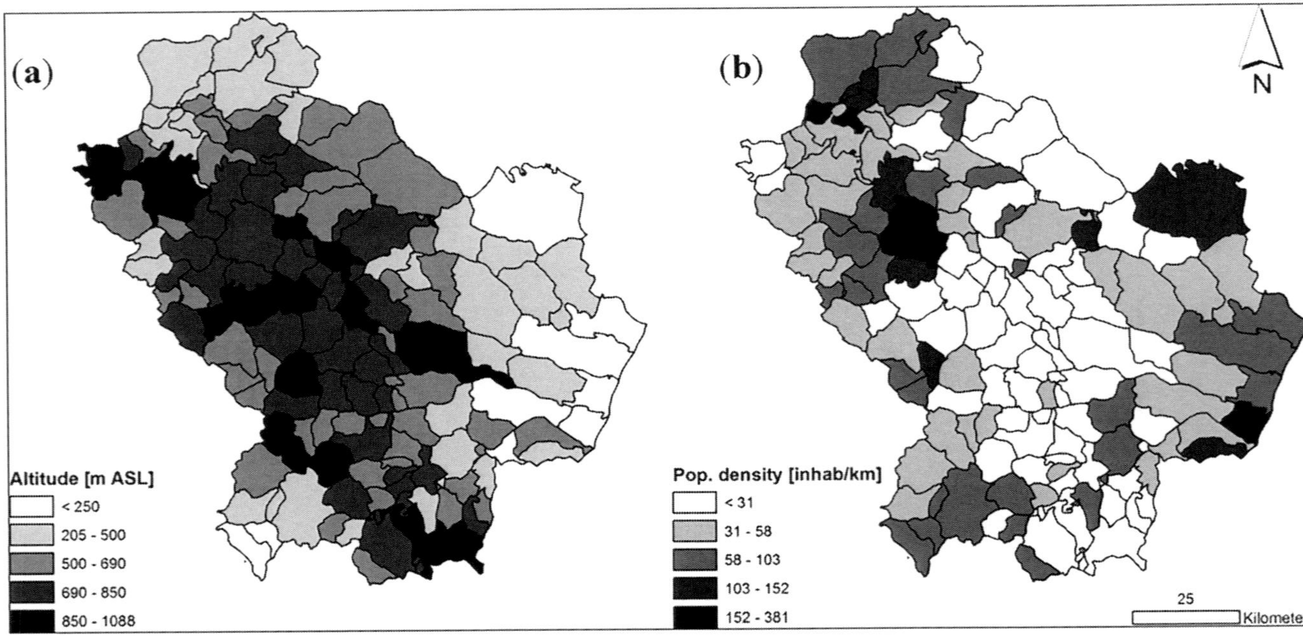

Figure 2. Average altitude (a) and population density (b) in Basilicata region.

below 3000 inhab with an average population density varying between 31 and 380 inhab km^{-2} (average: 57 inhab km^{-2}; Figure 2b).

The average MSW production (1.08 kg inhab^{-1} d^{-1}) is less than the national average [36,37]. During the last few years, a 2% y^{-1} increase in the MSW average production occurred, with peaks of 5% y^{-1} in the largest towns.

7.2.2 CHARACTERISTICS OF WASTE PRODUCTION

A survey was carried out with the aim of determining both the sieved waste composition and the influence on the combustible waste characteristics [37]. The mesh size was determined by considering that it has a considerable effect on the quantity of the obtainable energy [38].

Experimental tests were carried out on the waste collected in urban centers, with a production rate that fell in the range 0.8–1.2 kg inhab^{-1} d^{-1}. The percentages of separation by sieving were determined experimentally and the different product fraction percentages were deduced on the basis of the average composition of the waste. The data was determined as a function of the amount, in terms of weight, of the individual fractions of over-sieved (OS) and under-sieved (US) waste. This data can be extended to all compositions, on the assumption that if the amount, in terms of weight, of the single fraction is varied, the size does not change. Predictions in MSW evolution concerning quantity and composition were carried out considering: (i) past data; (ii) population growth; (iii) evolution of policies regarding separated collection [36].

The HV of each fraction was estimated using data found in scientific literature [32,39] (organic: 2,930.2 kJ kg^{-1}; paper: 12,558.0 kJ kg^{-1}; plastic and rubber: 20,930.0 kJ kg^{-1}; wood, textile and leather: 15,488.2 kJ kg^{-1}; under-sieved waste below 20 mm: 5,651.1 kJ kg^{-1}) and was applied to each OS fraction in order to obtain the respective energy content.

7.2.3 ENVIRONMENTAL EFFECTS ASSESSMENT

The GHGs emission assessment of three ISWM possible solution was carried out considering the influence of the sieve cut-off [40]. Such solutions

Table 1. Emission factors adopted for the environmental effects assessment.

	Treatment	GHGs emissions	
Biostabilization	without energy recovery	kg CH_4eq kg^{-1} biodegradable VSS	2.5
	with energy recovery		1.5
Incineration plant	50% of biodegradable fraction removal	kg CH_4eq kg^{-1} VSS	1.5
Landfilling (50% of biogas capture)	without energy recovery	kg CH_4eq kg^{-1} biodegradable VSS	10.5
	with energy recovery		9.5

are: (a) the direct MSW landfilling; (b) US landfilling and OS incineration; (c) US biostabilization and OS incineration. Table 1 reports the emission factors assumed for the environmental assessment [40,41].

7.2.4 MODELING

7.2.4.1 PROCESS AND MODEL DESCRIPTION

The combined production may be regarded as one of the best strategies for MSW management, in terms of efficiency, pollution and management costs [43–45]. The layout of the examined plant is shown in Figure 3.

The thermal cycle used for power recovery is composed of a gas turbine coupled with a water steam cycle, where the heat entering the steam cycle is obtained from the thermal recovery carried out on the gas turbine exhaust. Before being sent for treatment, the high-temperature combustion gases go through a heat exchanger, where heat is transferred, and what comes out is a liquid at a lower temperature. Then the heated and compressed air is sent to the gas turbine. The emitted gases are introduced into a steam generator. A mono-phase counter-pressure steam turbine was considered. The plant is completed by an electrical power generator and by the heat exchangers for producing hot water. Moreover, the plant includes a condensate collector, centrifuge pumps and a degasser for treating the condensate water and the steam. For the gas-gas heat exchanger a Ljungström-type rotating system [46] was used.

In the case of combustion under practical conditions (n > 1), the exhaust gas discharge is equal to:

$$m_f = m_{sw} - (m_{sg} + m_{fa}) + m_{ae}$$

In order to calculate the above terms, we used the following equations:

$$m_{sg} = \chi_{sg} \cdot m_{sw}$$

$$m_{fa} = \chi_{fa} \cdot m_{sw}$$

$$m_{at} = \chi_{at} \cdot m_{sw}$$

$$m_{ae} = n \cdot m_{at}$$

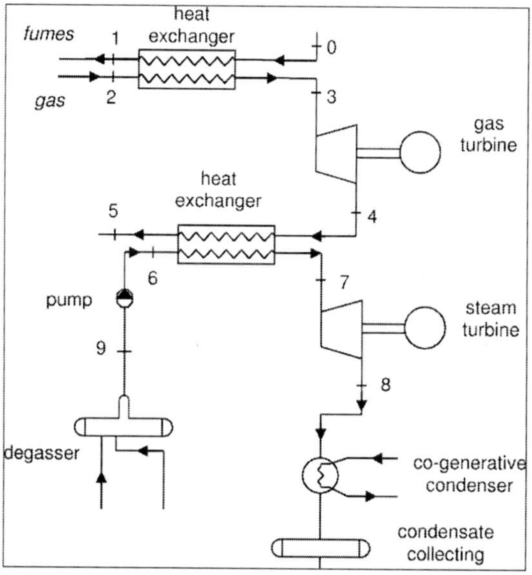

Figure 3. The examined combined cycle plant layout. Numbers indicates the calculation sections.

If there are no unburned substances, and no heat exchange between the gases and the combustion chamber, the gas temperature only depends on the fuel characteristics, the air index n as well as the initial air and fuel temperatures. In practice, a temperature T_f equal to the theoretical combustion temperature, T_{ad}, is considered:

$$T_{ad}=\tau+\frac{HV}{c_f\cdot(n\cdot m_{at})}$$

The temperature of the gas entering the turbine is given by the equation below, by accepting for the gas-gas exchanger an efficiency of $\varepsilon_{g\text{-}g}$:

$$T_3=T_2+\frac{\varepsilon_{g\text{-}g}(m_f\cdot c_f)\Delta T_{0\text{-}2}}{m_g\cdot c_g}$$

The temperature of the gas leaving the turbine, considering the 3-4 adiabatic transformation (Figure 3) as reversible, is given by the following equation:

$$T_4=T_3\cdot\beta^{(1-k)/k}$$

The electrical power, produced by the alternator coupled to the gas turbine, is given by the equation:

$$W_{GT}=\eta_{GT}\cdot(m_g\cdot c_{GT})\cdot\Delta T_{3\text{-}4}$$

With an efficiency of the air-water heat exchanger of $\varepsilon_{g\text{-}w}$, the steam discharge in the turbine is:

$$m_{ST}=\frac{(m_g c_{GT})\cdot\varepsilon_{g\text{-}w}\cdot\Delta T_{4\text{-}6}}{\Delta h_{7\text{-}6}}$$

Considering a total efficiency η_{ST} for the steam turbine section, the electrical power developed is:

$$W_{ST}=\eta_{ST}\cdot m_{ST}\cdot\Delta h_{7\text{-}8}$$

The steam/water heat exchanger operates with a gradient of ΔT_{7-6}.

The co-generated thermal energy is equal to:

$$Q = m_s \cdot \Delta h_{8-9}$$

A water discharge is transferred, and is equal to:

$$m_W = \frac{Q}{c_W \cdot \Delta T_{7-6}}$$

The first-principle yield of the co-generative combined cycle plant (η_I) is:

$$\eta_I = \frac{W_{ST} + W_{GT} + Q}{m_{sw} \cdot HV}$$

The yield is lower because a part of Q is wasted while it is transported to the heating.

In co-generative plants, we also consider a second-principle yield (η_{II}) which takes into account that the quantity of electrical power is much greater than the thermal power.

The analyzed energy is intended as the work, which can be obtained as a system returns to steady conditions. In the components of work production, the energy flow coincides with the electrical power; in the condenser, the energy flow is lower than the thermal flow because of the increase in the exchange fluid entropy. The available energy entering the plant coincides with the thermal power produced by the waste combustion. In the case of electricity generation only, η_{II} is equivalent to η_I. In the case of co-generation we have:

$$\eta_{II} = \frac{W_{ST} + W_{GT} + Q - (m_W \cdot T_W \cdot \Delta s)}{m_{sw} \cdot HV}$$

In order to use the waste heating value as a heating source for summer air-conditioning, we consider a value Y for the refrigeration yield; therefore we have:

$$\eta_{I summer} = \frac{W_{ST} + W_{GT} + Y \cdot Q_{sw}}{m_{sw} \cdot HV}$$

7.2.4.2 DATA AND ASSUMPTIONS

The waste-to-energy plant is:

- intended to produce power and low temperature heat for feeding a heating network;
- situated in a strategic area that can be reached from every town through the ordinary communication routes;
- provided with a landfill in order to reduce the transportation of residual waste (e.g., ash, slag).

The HV of the secondary fuel used in the incineration plant results from the MSW analysis. Table 2 shows the values of the parameters used in the calculation.

7.3 RESULTS AND DISCUSSION

7.3.1 WASTE PRODUCTION AND ENERGY POTENTIAL EVOLUTION

Figure 4 shows the estimation of waste production as a function of different percentages of separated waste collection.

In the next 25 years the MSW production will increase almost linearly, reaching values of 420 and 600 t y^{-1} considering, respectively, the optimistic (35%) and the pessimistic (7%) percentages of separated collection.

Concerning the current composition (Table 3, second column), the MSW production varies greatly. The amount of biodegradable organic waste is equal to about 0.350 kg $inhab^{-1}$ d^{-1}, while the maximum level of paper and plastic collection is 50% of the national average. In the next decade, Basilicata MSW production will be involved in quality variations which will be more remarkable than the quantity ones. Figure 5 shows the results of an estimation of the waste composition in the next 12 y.

A strong reduction of organic fraction (−7.6%), a light reduction of glass (−2.2%), a negligible variation of metals, a sensitive increase of pa-

Table 2. Parameters for combustion calculations.

	Paramater		Unit	Value
Coefficients	theoretical combustion air (m_{at}/m_{sw})		-	4.300
	air index (n)		-	2.300
Production rates	slag (χ_{sg})		kg kg^{-1}	0.055
	flying ash (χ_{fa})		kg kg^{-1}	0.188
Specific heats	gases		kJ kg^{-1}K^{-1}	1.260
	gas entering the turbine		kJ kg^{-1}K^{-1}	1.009
	gas leaving the turbine		kJ kg^{-1}K^{-1}	1.165
	steam entering the turbine		kJ kg^{-1}K^{-1}	1.091
Yield	heat exchanger	gas-gas (ε_{g-g})	-	0.950
		gas-water(ε_{g-w})	-	0.700
	Turbine	gas-fed	-	0.730
		steam-fed	-	0.730
	refrigerating machine (Y)		-	0.800

The combustion gas temperature, T_f, is 95 °C.

pers and plastics (+8.8% and +8.6%, respectively) and a light increase of wood and textiles (+0.5%) will occur.

Table 3 reports the data relative to the percentage composition of the OS MSW. About half of the waste is smaller than 60 mm and less than 20% is composed by the fine fraction (<20 mm). The composition of the oversized fraction (>120 mm) largely depends on the high HV materials (plastic, paper and textiles), while the major part of the organic fraction is below 60 mm. Glass and inert matter have a homogeneous distribution.

Table 4 shows the HV of separated waste as a function of the sieve size.

Considering the HV as a function of the MSW sieve cut-off, the trend is almost linear: the energy content of the fine fraction is about 64% of the oversized fraction (>120 mm).

7.3.2 MODELING

7.3.2.1 ENVIRONMENTAL EFFECTS

Figure 6 shows the GHGs emissions for three proposed ISWM solutions.

As expected, the solution with direct landfilling (solution a) generates the highest emissions (e.g., biomethane). In areas where a low waste production occurs (such as Basilicata), the effect is more evident because of the long residence times of waste before the landfill closure and the biogas extraction network completion. The direct US landfilling coupled with OS incineration (solution b) generates more GHGs when the amount of burned MSW diminishes. The sieve cut-off influences also landfill volumes uses and energy recovery. In fact, smaller is the sieve cut-off (20–40 mm), the higher is the waste volume reduction; conversely, higher is the sieve cut-off (60–80 mm), the lower is the waste volume reduction and the higher is

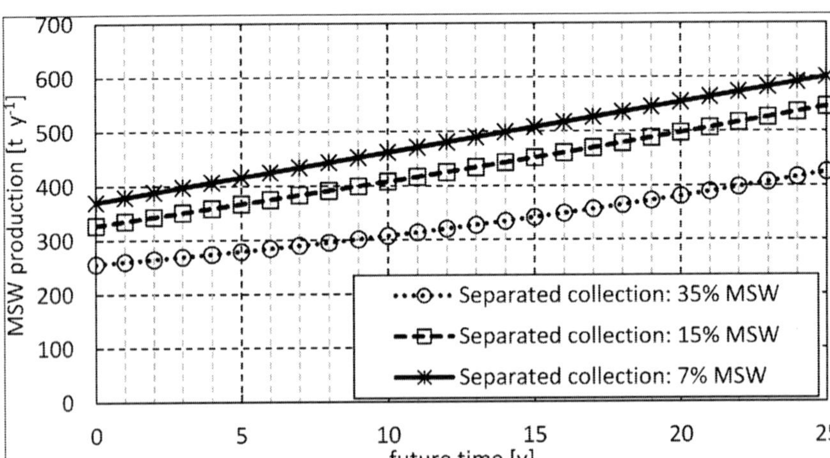

Figure 4. Waste production trend as a function of separated waste collection.

the energy recovery. The separation of the wet fraction, which is first aerobically stabilized in reactors and later disposed of in landfills (solution c) is the best solution, independently from the sieve cut-off; moreover, it allows to decrease the incineration unit size (theoretically, partly penalizing the potential energy recovery). We must also take into account that this phase will be gradually reduced by successively boosting of home composting.

7.3.2.2 WASTE INCINERATION AND ENERGY RECOVERY

According to an optimization procedure which considers a compromise between the environmental impact (GHG emissions) and the energy recovery, the sieve cut-off was set equal to 60 mm, corresponding to an HV equal to about 10.1 MJ kg^{-1} (Table 4).

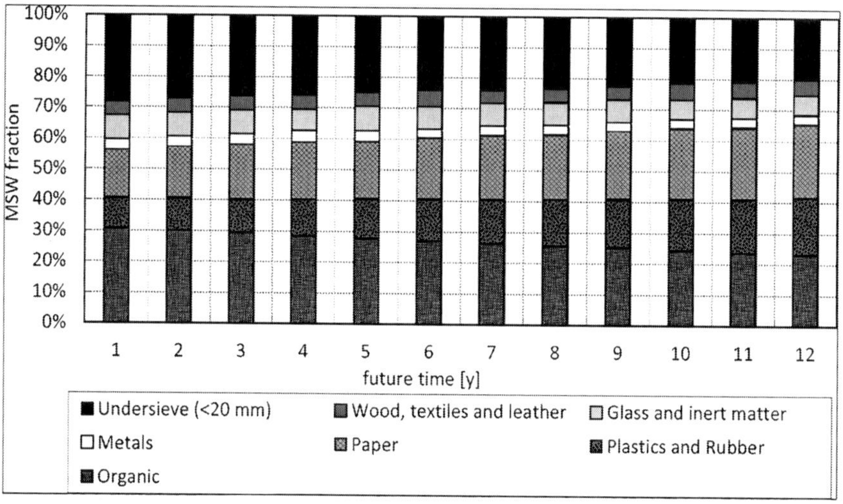

Figure 5. Estimation of the MSW composition in Basilicata.

Table 3. Percentage composition of both raw and over-sieved (OS) MSW.

MSW fraction	Raw MSW	Sieve cut-off (mm)				
		40	60	80	100	120
Organic	34.3	70.3	39.6	24.3	13.3	6.4
Paper	20.5	96.1	83.5	77.7	69.1	59.4
Plastic and rubber	11.4	93.5	83.2	81.3	73.9	63.4
Wood, textile and leather	5.4	85.3	70.3	63.7	61.9	59.8
Glass and inert matter	6.6	89.7	67.1	50.3	32.4	15.8
Metals	3.0	88.3	82.9	73.3	57.9	49.3
Under-sieved (20 mm)	18.8	-	-	-	-	-
Total	100.0	67.6	50.9	42.5	34.4	27.4

Table 4. Heating value (in kJ kg^{-1}) of the over-sieved MSW fraction.

MSW fraction	Raw MSW	Sieve cut-off (mm)					
		20	40	60	80	100	120
Organic	1,004.0	1,236.6	1,043.4	781.1	574.1	388.4	234.8
Paper	2,576.0	3,172.9	3,659.7	4,225.7	4,709.7	5,177.5	5,591.8
Plastic and rubber	2,378.2	2,929.2	3,287.3	3,887.2	4,549.6	5,112.0	5,510.1
Wood, textile and leather	840.2	1,034.9	1,059.6	1,160.4	1,259.4	1,512.9	1,836.2
Glass and inert matter	-	-	-	-	-	-	-
Metals	-	-	-	-	-	-	-
Under-sieved	5,651.1	1,063.1	-	-	-	-	-
Total	6,861.4	8,373.6	9,050.0	10,054.4	11,092.8	12,190.8	13,172.9

For the gas-gas heat exchanger, the discharge is $m_{GT} = 1.3\ m_f$ ($m_f = 60$ kg s^{-1}) using a gas temperature in the turbine, T_3 equal to 884 °C. The operating conditions of the gas turbine are: entry pressure of 9.1 kPa; pressure ratio (β) equal to 7.1. The entry temperature and pressure into the turbine are 60 bar and 440 °C, respectively. At the output, there is an optimum level for operation of the turbine, which is no lower than 0.9, and a temperature of approximately 100 °C. With a steam discharge equal to 8.4 kg s^{-1}, the power produced by the alternator coupled with the gas turbine is 25.1 MW. The power developed by the steam turbine is 5.4 MW with a gradient that can be used to produce 30 °C hot water. The co-generated thermal power, Q, is 16.8 MW, which is transferred to a water flow, mw, of 200 kg s^{-1}.

The second-principle yield (η_{II}), in the case of power generation only, is 0.47, while the first- and second-principle yields related to co-generation are 0.74 and 0.54, respectively. In the case of a demand for cold air (used for summer conditioning), η_I summer is 0.68. Therefore, the results show a co-generation second-principle yield lower than η_I because of the difference between the thermal power to the condenser and the electrical power, but higher than η_I in the case of electrical generation only. The major advantage associated with the co-generation respect to the power production must be compared to the higher costs of plant start-up and maintenance.

In the urban area of Potenza (the main town in Basilicata), the locations of the waste disposal, incineration and treatment plants aid the implementation of an interconnection system aimed at energy recovery. Thus, the best solution for the examined case is the integrated management of the energy sources, which entails (i) using the MSW combustible fraction; (ii) managing the landfill and (iii) stabilizing the wastewater treatment plant sludge. In fact, the thermal energy necessary for heating the anaerobic reactors as well as for evaporating percolates and digested sludge can be satisfied by cogeneration plant. Moreover, during summer, when cold is demanded for air-conditioning, it is possible to use an absorption refrigeration cycle, albeit such solution implies an increase in plant costs.

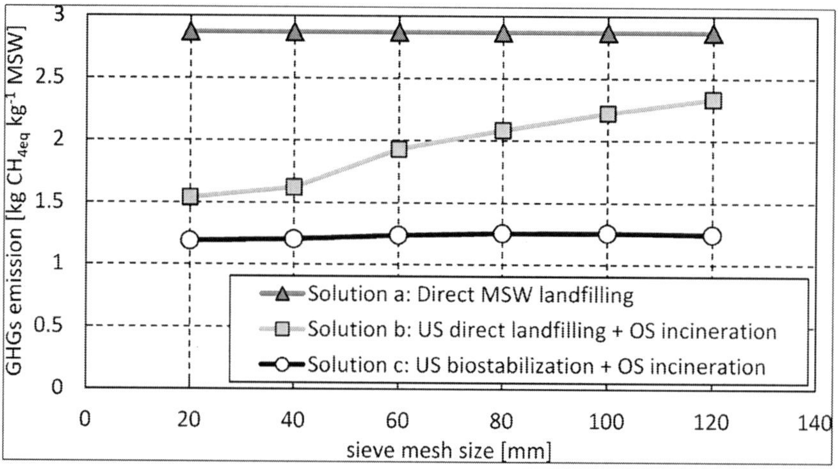

Figure 6. Greenhouse gases (GHGs) emissions for different integrated solid waste management (ISWM) solutions.

7.4 CONCLUSIONS

The rapid increase in volume and composition of MSW as a result of continuous economic growth, urbanization and industrialization is a problem for national and local governments, if they aim at ensuring an effective and sustainable management of waste. Solid waste incineration requires complex and sophisticated plants, whose running and installation costs are much higher than those of plants that work with traditional fuels. Moreover, energy recovery in fairly small-sized plants is affected by the high cost of the interventions.

The paper focuses on non-densely populated area where the production of urban waste is less than the urban ones. Considering the difficulties in waste collection due to geographic and demographic conditions, separated collection should be carried out only for complying with the regulations. The residual fraction should be sent to the incineration process for energy recovery, with positive environmental effects (in terms of GHGs emissions and landfill volumes) for the whole ISWM system.

Moreover, in low waste production area where the establishment of a unique MSW collection policy is difficult, the residual fraction quality is variable. Such issue can be solved with an appropriate pre-treatment process which improves the characteristics (e.g., heating value) of secondary fuel. The analysis of the obtained results in an Italian non-densely populated area demonstrates the potential of the co-generative incineration residual MSW for energy recovery after sieving, an effective and low cost pre-treatment process. Co-generative incineration is advantageous from an energetic point of view, especially considering the quality and the amount of the energy that can be obtained (power, heat and/or cold).

All these factors, including also the European regulations constraint and the low cost of secondary fuel which tends to increase its heating value, should be taken into account for a sustainable mid-term ISWM system planning in both developing and developed countries where the sustainable management of MSW cycle is penalized by the difficulties in source separated collection and the low flow of material recovery.

REFERENCES

1. United Nations—U.N. Environment Programme. Developing Integrated Solid Waste Management Plan; Training Manual; International Environmental Technology Centre: Osaka/Shiga, Japan, 2009; Volume 4.
2. Cossu, R.; Masi, S. Re-thinking incentives and penalties: Economic aspects of waste management in Italy. Waste Manag. 2013, 33, 2541–2547.
3. Callegari, A.; Torretta, V.; Capodaglio, A.G. Preliminary trial application of biological desulfonation in pig farms' anaerobic digesters. Environ. Eng. Manag. 2013, 12, 815–819.
4. Rada, E.C.; Ragazzi, M.; Torretta, V. Laboratory-scale anaerobic sequencing batch reactor for treatment of stillage from fruit distillation. Water Sci. Technol. 2013, 67, 1068–1074.
5. Martinez, S.L.; Torretta, V.; Minguela, J.V.; Siñeriz, F.; Raboni, M.; Copelli, S.; Rada, E.C.; Ragazzi, M. Treatment of slaughterhouse wastewaters using anaerobic filters. Environ. Technol. 2013, doi:10.1080/09593330.2013.827729.

6. Torretta, V.; Rada, E.C.; Istrate, I.A.; Ragazzi, M. Poultry manure gasification and its energy yield. UPB-Sci. Bull. Ser. D 2013, 75, 231–238.
7. Vaccari, M.; Torretta, V.; Collivignarelli, C. Effect of improving environmental sustainability in developing countries by upgrading solid waste management techniques: A case study. Sustainability 2012, 4, 2852–2861.
8. Hartmann, H.; Ahring, B.K. Anaerobic digestion of the organic fraction of municipal solid waste: Influence of co-digestion with manure. Water Res. 2005, 39, 1543–1552.
9. Chaerul, M.; Tnaka, M. A system dynamics approach for hospital waste management. Waste Manag. 2008, 28, 442–449.
10. Birpmar, M.E.; Bilgili, M.S.; Erdoğan,T. Medical waste management in Turkey: A case study of Istanbul. Waste Manag. 2009, 29, 445–448.
11. Abdulla, F.; Abu Qdais, H.; Rabi, A. Site investigation on medical waste management practices in northern Jordan. Waste Manag. 2008, 28, 450–458.
12. Mancini, G.; Tamma, R.; Viotti, P. Thermal process of fluff: Preliminary tests on a full-scale treatment plant. Waste Manag. 2010, 30, 1670–1682.
13. Torretta, V.; Istrate, I.; Rada, E.C.; Ragazzi, M. Management of waste electrical and electronic equipment in two EU countries: A comparison. Waste Manag. 2013, 33, 117–122.
14. Di Mauro, C.; Bouchon, S.; Torretta, V. Industrial risk in the Lombardy Region (Italy): What people perceive and what are the gaps to improve the risk communication and the partecipatory processes. Chem. Eng. Trans. 2012, 26, 297–302.
15. Morris, M.W.; Su, S.K. Social psychological obstacles in environmental conflict resolution. Am. Behav. Sci. 1999, 42, 1322–1349.
16. European Council. Directive 91/156/EEC Amending Directive 75/442/EEC on Waste; Official Journal L 078, 26/03/1991 P. 0032 – 0037; EEC: Brussels, Belgium, 1991.
17. European Council. Directive 91/689/EEC on Hazardous Waste; Official Journal L 377, 31/12/1991 P. 0020 – 0027; EEC: Brussels, Belgium, 1991.
18. European Parliament and Council. Directive 94/62/EC on Packaging and Packaging Waste; Official Journal L 365, 31/12/1994, P. 0010–0023; EC: Brussels, Belgium, 1994.
19. European Parliament and Council. Directive 2000/76/EC on the Incineration of Waste; Official Journal L 332, 28/12/2000, P. 0091; EC: Brussels, Belgium, 2000.
20. Italian Parliament. Decreto Legislativo 5 febbraio 1997, n. 22 —Attuazione delle direttive 91/156/CEE sui rifiuti, 91/689/CEE sui rifiuti pericolosi e 94/62/CE sugli imballaggi e sui rifiuti di imballaggio‖. Available online: http://www.parlamento.it/parlam/leggi/deleghe/97022dl.htm (accessed on 2 May 2013).
21. Italian Parliament. Decreto Legislativo 3 aprile 2006, n. 152 —Norme in materia ambientale‖. Available online: http://www.camera.it/parlam/leggi/deleghe/06152dl.htm (accessed on 2 May 2013).
22. Eriksson, O.; Carlsson, R.M.; Frostell, B.; Björklund, A.; Assefa, G.; Sundquist, J.-O.; Granath, J.; Baky, A.; Thyselius, L. Municipal solid waste management from a systems perspective. J. Clean. Prod. 2005, 13, 241–252.
23. Tascione, V.; Raggi, A. Identification and selection of alternative scenarios in LCA studies of integrated waste management systems: A review of main issues and perspectives. Sustainability 2012, 4, 2430–2442.

24. Bovea,M.D.;Ibáñez-Forés,V.;Gallardo,A.;Colomer-Mendoza,F.J.Environmentalass essment of alternative municipal solid waste management strategies: A Spanish case study. Waste Manag. 2010, 30, 2383–2395.
25. De Feo, G.; Malvano, C. The use of LCA in selecting the best MSW management system. Waste Manag. 2009, 29, 1901–1915.
26. Iriarte,A.;Gabarrel,X.;Rieradevall,J.LCAofselectivewastecollectionsystemsin-denseurban areas. Waste Manag. 2009, 29, 903–914.
27. Emery, A.; Davies, A.; Griffiths, A.; Williams, K. Environmental and economic modelling: A case study of municipal solid waste management scenarios in Wales. Resour. Conserv. Recycl. 2007, 49, 244–263.
28. Chang, Y.H.; Chang, N.B. Compatibility analysis of material and energy recovery in a regional solid waste management system. J. Air Waste Manag. Assoc. 2003, 53, 32–40.
29. Di Maria, F.; Micale, C. Impact of source segregation intensity of solid waste on fuel consumption and collection costs. Waste Manag. 2013, 33, 2170–2176.
30. Nguyen, T.T.T.; Wilson, B.G. Fuel consumption estimation for kerbside municipal solid waste (MSW) collection activities. Waste Manag. Res. 2010, 28, 289–297.
31. European Commission. Eurostat Database. Available online: http://epp.eurostat.ec.europa.eu/ portal/page/portal/statistics/search_database (accessed on 1 December 2013).
32. Tchobanoglous,G.; Kreith, F. Handbook of Solid Waste Management; McGraw-Hill: New York, NY, USA, 2002.
33. Murphy, J.D.; McKeogh, E. Technical, economic and environmental analysis of energy production from municipal solid waste. Renew. Energy 2004, 29, 1043–1057.
34. Rimaitytė, I.; Denafas, G.; Martuzevicius, D.; Kavaliauskas, A. Energy and environmental indicators of municipal solid waste incineration: Toward selection of an optimal waste management system. Pol. J. Environ. Stud. 2010, 19, 989–998.
35. Italian Institute of Statistics (ISTAT), Maps and Census Data (in Italian). Available online: http://www.istat.it/it/strumenti/cartografia (accessed on 23 April 2013).
36. Institute for the Environmental Protection and Research—ISPRA. Rapporto rifiuti urbani (Municipal Waste Report); ISRRA: Rome, Italy, 2012.
37. Regione Basilicata. Piano regionale gestione rifiuti, Potenza, Italy. Available online: http://www.regione.basilicata.it/giunta/files/docs/DOCUMENT_FILE_242375.pdf (accessed on 20 April 2013).
38. Consonni,S.;Viganò,F.Materialandenergyrecoveryinintegratedwastemanagement-systems: The potential for energy recovery. Waste Manag. 2011, 31, 2074–2084.
39. Valkenburg, C.; Gerber, M.A.; Walton, C.W.; Jones, S.B.; Thompson, B.L.; Stevens, D.J. Municipal Solid Waste (MSW) to Liquid Fuels Synthesis, Volume 1: Availability of Feedstock and Technology; U.S. Deptartment of Energy: Washington, DC, USA, 2008.
40. Cosmi,C.;Cuomo,V.;Macchiato,M.;Mangiamele,L.;Masi,S.;Salvia,M.Wasteman-agement modeling by MARKAL model: A case study for Basilicata Region. Environ. Model. Assess. 2000, 5, 19–27.
41. Cosmi,C.;Mancini,I.;Mangiamele,L.;Masi,S.;Salvia,M.;Macchiato,M.Themanage-mentof urban waste at regional scale: The state of the art and its strategic evolu-

tion—Case study Basilicata Region (Southern Italy). Fresenius Environ. Bull. 2001, 10, 131–138.

42. Çengel, Y. A. Introduction to Thermodynamics and Heat Transfer; McGraw-Hill: New York, NY, USA, 2007.
43. Environmental Protection Agency—Ireland. Municipal Solid Waste—Pre-treatment & Residuals Management; IR-EPA: Wexford, Ireland, 2009.
44. Sue, D.C.; Chuang, C.C. Engineering design and energy analyses for combustion gas turbine based power generation system. Energy 2004, 29, 1183–1205.
45. Roher, A. Comparison of combined heat and power generation plants. ABB Review 1996, 3, 24–32.
46. Lombardi, F.; Lategano, E.; Cordiner, S.; Torretta, V. Waste incineration in rotary kilns: A new simulation combustion's tool to support design and technical change. Waste Manag. Res. 2013, 31, 739–750.

PART IV

WATER MANAGEMENT

CHAPTER 8

Innovative Urban Water Management as a Climate Change Adaptation Strategy: Results from the Implementation of the Project "Water Against Climate Change (WATACLIC)"

GIULIO CONTE, ANDREA BOLOGNESI, CRISTIANA BRAGALLI, SARA BRANCHINI, ALESSANDRO DE CARLI, CHIARA LENZI, FABIO MASI, ANTONIO MASSARUTTO, MARCO POLLASTRI, AND ILARIA PRINCIPI

8.1 INTRODUCTION

The excessive use of water is damaging European groundwater and rivers: their environmental conditions are often below the "good status" that—according to the Water Framework Directive 2000/60—should be reached by 2015 [1]. In Italy the situation is still critical: more than 50% of the river water quality sampling stations in 2010 did not reach the "good status" (Table 1).

The already critical situation is tending to get worse because of climate change. According to IPCC [3] and EU [4], one of the most important effects of Climate Change concerns water: beside the risk of more uneven precipitation patterns throughout the continent, an increase of dry periods is predicted especially in the southern part of Europe. In the coming years, therefore, several European areas, already experiencing water stress—such as Greece, Southern Italy and Spain—will evolve towards more severe conditions (Figure 1).

High water abstraction is a major problem in Mediterranean countries, where a reduction of water use—especially in the water intensive sector of agriculture—is absolutely needed in order to increase natural water flow in rivers and groundwater [5]. In Southern Europe, then, a sustainable water management approach should combine efficient water use in all sectors, together with a reduction of pollution loads due to urban wastewater along with industrial and agriculture sources. However, even in water rich countries, such as those in Northern Europe, urban wastewater is still one of the main sources of water pollution: wastewater treatment performance would benefit highly from a reduction in domestic water use (biological

Table 1. River water quality in Italy, year 2010. Water quality classification according to EU Directive 2000/60 criteria; Data from ISPRA [2].

Geographical area	Very good %	Good %	Sufficient %	Poor %	Very poor %	Sampling stations
Northern Italy	11	58	24	7	0	131
Central Italy	4	38	35	16	7	246
Southern Italy	3	32	43	19	3	172
Italy	6	40	35	15	4	549

treatment processes are concentration limited: the lower the concentration of the treatment inflow, the larger the pollution load at the effluent after treatment). Currently, urban soil sealing and "conventional" rainwater management, planned to quickly move rainwater away from roofs and streets, are increasing the flood risk.

In Italy, besides the irrigation sector (responsible for more than 25 billion of water withdrawal, 50% of the country's water use), the excessive use of water concerns urban water use. From 1987 to 2008 water withdrawal for urban use increased by more than 1 billion m^3 (cubic meters), exceeding nine billion m^3 of yearly withdrawal (Figure 2), while the per capita daily consumption of water delivered to households, even though slightly decreasing, is amongst the highest in Europe (more than 0.25 m^3/inhabitant/day) [7].

Thus urban water use in Italy is affected by two major problems. First, the excess of water withdrawal: due to the poor performance of the distribution network nearly 40% of water withdrawn is lost on the way and does not reach the final users. The problem has become worse in recent times: that is why in 2008 the total water volume withdrawn increased, while the volume delivered decreased. Secondly, the high per capita water consumption and, consequently, the dilution of the wastewater collected (BOD5 concentration is very often below 150 mg/L), affect the pollution removal capacity of the treatment plants, which usually work better when more concentrated liquids are to be treated. Moreover, the "centralised" wastewater treatment approach adopted in past decades results in the discharge of huge mass fluxes at a single point. Thus, even the outflows which respect legal concentration limits, discharge at a very large flow rate and, consequently, contain a large amount of pollutants. Whenever the receiving water flow is unable to dilute the treatment plant effluents, such as during summer low flows, most river stretches located downstream do not meet the WFD 2000/60 quality standards for "good status".

What is even more surprising is that the high per capita consumption is not perceived as a problem, either by the public, or by water service operators, who in their provisional plans expect to increase the water volume for distribution for urban use by 2020 (Table 2).

Water Authorities do not comprehend the need of more rational water use: a recent report [8] carried out for the Italian Government by the as-

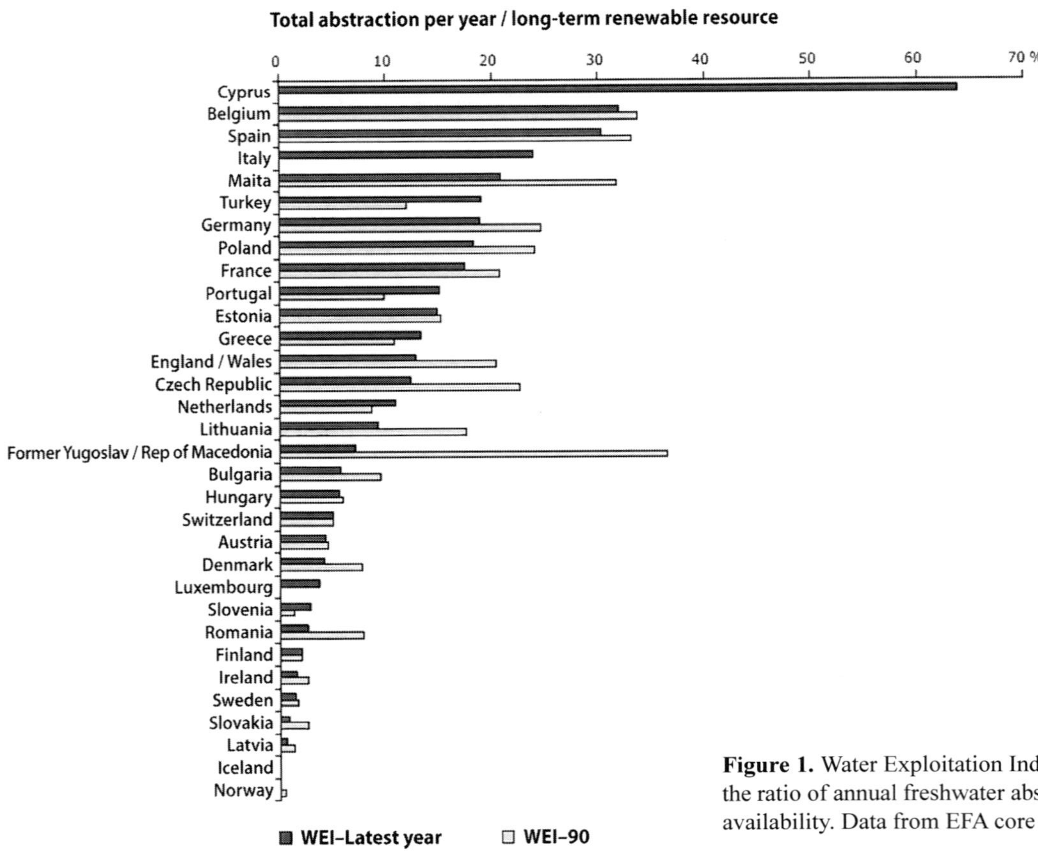

Figure 1. Water Exploitation Index in EU countries. WEI is the ratio of annual freshwater abstraction to long-term water availability. Data from EFA core set indicator 018 [6].

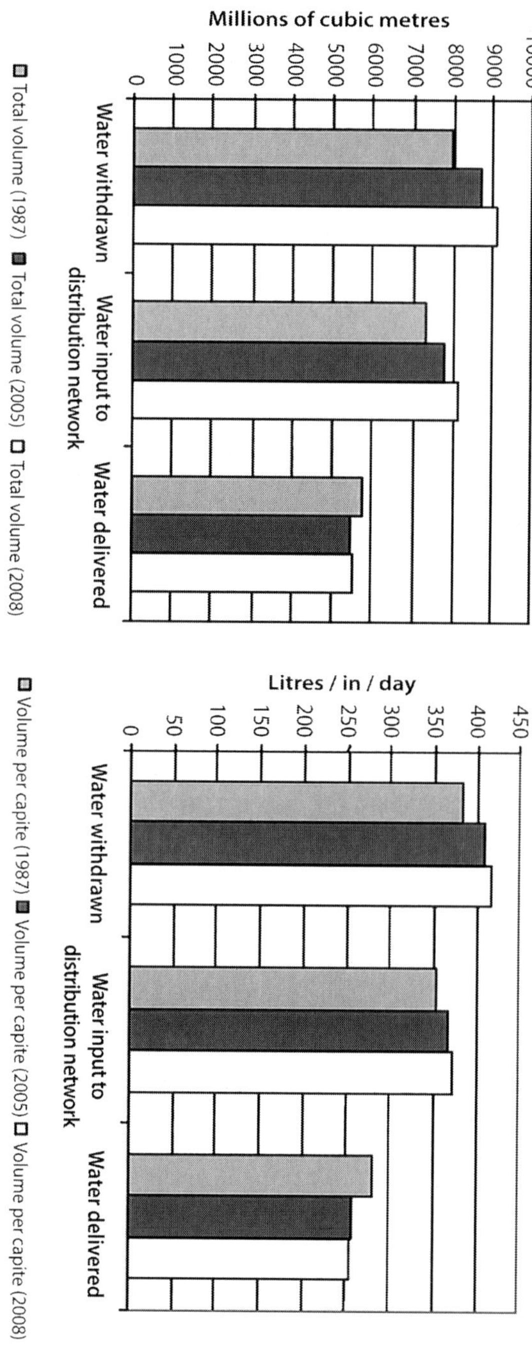

Figure 2. Water withdrawal and consumption for urban use in Italy. Data are from ISTAT [7].

Table 2. Expected water volume distributed in Italy for urban use (millions of m^3) [8].

Geographical area	2010	2011	2012	2015	2020
North-West	1681	1683	1685	1693	1706
Nord-East	1165	1168	1171	1182	1194
Centre	1010	1012	1014	1019	1027
South	1141	1149	1156	1174	1190
Islands	573	584	596	606	614
Italy	5570	5596	5622	5674	5731

sociation of water management companies, states: "Data from Water Plans clearly show—contrary to what is asked by the European Water Framework Directive—an increasing trend in water demand, clearly showing the Italian difficulties to conform to the EU policy orientation". Similarly, the need to reduce water consumption at household level is not widely perceived by the various stakeholders.

There are several causes of the present situation of water management in Italy: the most important being the lack of knowledge about new approaches of sustainable water management. Technical and administrative operators of the water sector, having been trained to operate the water service with the sole aim of satisfying final users, have very little knowledge of the availability of new technical, financial and communication tools able to bring households towards a more sustainable water use. Another important aspect concerns the water cost, that in Italy, according to Global Water Intelligence [9] is among the lowest in Europe, ranging between 0.50 and 2.50 €/m^3. However the situation does vary throughout the country and recent data shows that water consumption is higher where cost is lower (Figure 3).

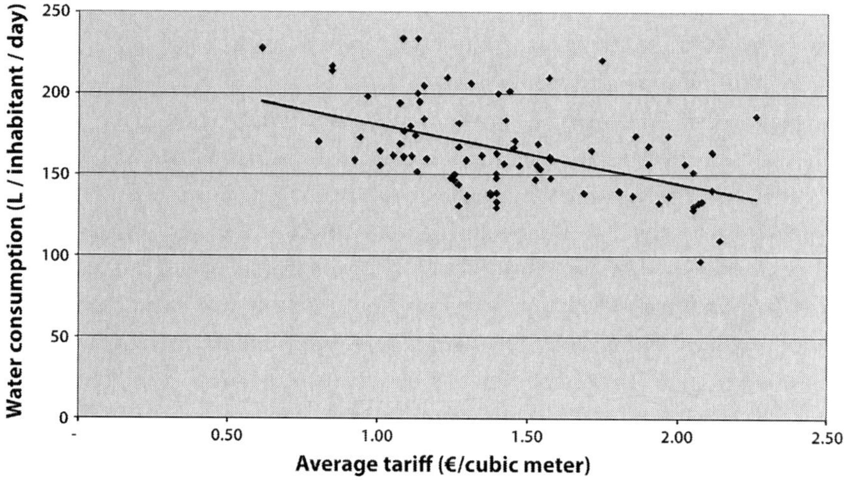

Figure 3. Trend of water consumption related to water tariffs in main Italian cities. Elaboration of the authors on data from ISTAT [7].

8.2 METHODOLOGY: WATACLIC—AN INFORMATION AND COMMUNICATION PROJECT TO DISSEMINATE BEST PRACTICE

As recently recognized by the European Environmental Agency "to prevent urban water crises, we need to manage water resources effectively at every stage: from the supply of clean water to its different uses by the consumers. This could involve reducing consumption as well as finding new ways of collecting and using water. Water management should also be better integrated within wider urban management while taking into account characteristics of the local environment" [10].

In this context Sustainable Water Management (SWM) technologies and approaches would allow a reduction of water abstraction and wastewater production while improving urban hydrological response to heavy rains [11]. Different kinds of SWM solutions can be adopted by final users or by water service operators. They range from very simple technologies—such as flow reduction tools for taps and showers or low flushing toilets—to the use of alternative water sources (rain water or treated greywater) for nondrinkable uses [12,13], to urine separation and dry sanitation equipment [14,15], to pressure management and water loss control in the distribution network [16,17], to the large "family" of SUDS (Sustainable Urban Drainage Systems) [18].

When the WATACLIC project was conceived, back in 2008, the question was: How can such technologies and approaches be promoted throughout Europe, and specifically in Italy? Information and communication tools play a strategic role for innovation in the field of urban and domestic water management. Moreover sustainable water management practices and approaches concern not only technicians who operate the water services, but also other stakeholders: public administrators, NGOs, households, and plumbers. The objective of WATACLIC is to provide proper information to different key stakeholders to promote innovative approaches to urban water management in order to disseminate culture and technologies through specific campaigns focussed on different target audiences: bodies in charge of water planning and management, urban planners, local authorities, the toilet and sanitation manufacture industry, and the building sector. After the creation of a database of SWM technologies (more than 60 records) and good practice experiences (18 records), five different information campaigns were conceived (refer to Table 3 for more information on these activities). Each campaign envisaged that workshops be organized by WATACLIC partners (Ambiente Italia, IRIDRA, the Universities of Bologna and Udine, Centro Antartide, the NGO that manages the national website on water saving) together with local partners (regional governments, local authorities, universities and research centres, and NGOs). The five campaigns had different target audiences:

- Water and Rules—Local authorities and urban planners: what solutions can be applied and how to promote them through urban planning and building regulations.
- Water and Money—Water authorities: water tariffs and other economic tools to discourage excessive use of drinking water and to promote innovative solutions; how to ensure social equality and not to penalize large households, assuring, in the meantime, financial feasibility of water services and investments.

Table 3. Summary of information activity of the WATACLIC project

Campaign	Target audience	Information contents	Responsible
Water and rules	Local Authorities and urban planners	Best practices of urban planning to promote: Rainwater harvesting; Greywater separation and re-use; Decentralised wastewater treatment systems (constructed wetlands); Sustainable urban drainage systems (SUDS)	Ambiente Italia & IRIDRA
Water and money	Water Authorities	Tariffing systems, economic incentives in water policy	University of Udine
Water and energy	Water and wastewater management utilities	Leakage detection, pressure control, pumping optimization, micro energy production plants	University of Bologna
Water and citizens	Public Administrations, Utilities and NGOs	Effective information campaigns: target, timing, old and new media, monitoring	Università Verde di Bologna
Water and innovation	Industry and plumbing service enterprises	Water saving (tap aerators, low flush toilets, etc.), rainwater harvesting and re-use, segregation and re-use of greywater	Ambiente Italia & IRIDRA

- Water and Energy—Water and wastewater management utilities: innovative solutions to reduce water losses and improve the energy efficiency of water services.
- Water and Citizens—Public administrations, utilities and NGOs: conception of effective information campaigns in order to encourage consumers to adopt a more responsible behavior towards water consumption and to use technologies that improve water and energy efficiency (low consumption sanitation devices and home appliances).
- Water and Innovation—Industry and plumbing service enterprises: disseminate knowledge and technologies for sustainable water management with regard to domestic plumbers.

8.3 PROJECT RESULTS

Apparently, in Italy water is not a very "trendy" issue. Involvement of the target audiences in WATACLIC campaigns has proved to be quite difficult: more events than originally planned have been organized in order to reach a satisfactory number of participants. In addition interviews with the participants showed a general, low-medium level of knowledge of the themes discussed during the workshops as well as difficulties in adopting the proposed measures and approaches in their professional activities (Table 4, gives an example of interviews for two of the campaigns).

Campaigns that showed higher participation rates (Table 5) were: water and money, confirming the existing awareness on the economic issues,

Table 4. The results of most of the information from questionnaires that participants were asked to fill in before the events of the campaigns; Water and Rules and Water and Money. Answers are given on a 1(lowest)–5 (highest) scale.

Themes	State of knowledge on the proposed themes	Interest in the proposed themes	Interest in adopting the proposed strategies
Techniques to reduce rainwater in sewage	2.4	3.7	3.8
Decentralized treatment systems (isolated neighborhoods, spillways)	2.2	3.6	3.6
Water saving and re-use	3.0	4.3	4.2
Integration of water management principles in building regulations	2.3	4.0	3.9
Different tariff structures and their effect to reach environmental, economic, financial and social goals	3.4	4.5	3.3
Financial instruments for urban water services in Italy and in other countries	3.5	4.4	3.4
Tools for territorial and social equality	2.9	4.0	3.2

and water and energy, the most "technical" one, targeted to a very specialized audience. Water and citizens and water and innovation had the worst participation performance. The low participation in events focusing on information campaigns water and citizens is maybe due to the sharp reduction of funds for communication activities linked to the recent financial crisis. However, more significant is the lack of interest on the issue by professional plumbers (water and innovation) who apparently do not identify domestic water saving innovative technologies as a profitable sector for their day-to-day work. The high number of participants in the water and rules campaign is mainly due to the high number of students participating in the two special events organized with technical and scientific institutions (universities, professional associations and bodies). The latter demonstrating an increasing interest of students and academic institutions in the themes proposed.

The project concept claimed that a significant decrease of water abstraction for urban use in Italy could be obtained by introducing the "WATACLIC" concepts in the ordinary activities of the targeted entities. More specifically the project objectives were the following:

- To introduce new rules in urban planning to help the diffusion among final users of technologies/strategies such as rainwater harvesting, greywater recycling and other techniques able to allow more sustainable urban water use.
- To adopt tariff schemes aimed at discouraging unwise use of water.
- To increase global efficiency (in terms of water and energy consumptions) of water supply systems.
- To adopt more effective awareness raising campaigns directed at the general public.
- To improve knowledge and awareness of plumber professional organization concerning water saving techniques.
- To emphasize the link between water use and energy consumption.

Have such objectives been reached?

Table 5. The results of the campaigns in terms of participants. Note that students who attended the events are not included in "participating entities" but only in "participants".

Campaign	Participating entities			Participants		
	Achieved	Expected	Result (%)	Achieved	Expected	Result (%)
Water and Rules	303	400	76%	661	500	132%
Water and Money	117	80	146%	250	-	-
Water and Citizens	109	150	73%	177	-	-
Water and Energy	155	75	207%	286	-	-
Water and Innovation	-	-	-	50	60	83%
Total	684	705	97%	1424	560	127%

8.3.1 NEW URBAN RULES

In Italy, according to the report produced by the ONRE (National Observatory on Municipal Building Regulations) of Legambiente and CRESME (Economical, Sociological and Market Research Center), referring to data from 2011, 530 of the 8092 Italian Municipalities already include in their building regulation, rules on sustainable water management. The very large part—more than 90%—of them have new regulations, approved after the year 2005. In the coming years the building regulations of all the remaining Municipalities will be progressively updated and—considering also the need to fulfill the requirements of the new Climate Change Adaptation Plans—hopefully they will include the sustainable water management new rules. WATACLIC is playing a significant role in driving such a process by its "water and rules" campaign: 45 Municipalities of the 59 that participated in the events are not listed in the ONRE Report, and several professional experts who participated in the campaign will work in the coming years with other Municipalities to renew their regulations. A few important Provinces also participated in the Water and Rules events: among them Vicenza, Mantova and Rome are willing to publish guidelines for their Municipalities to urge them to include sustainable water management rules. Moreover, the success of the WATACLIC website—where all project materials are downloadable—in the past months (the number of accesses grew from 2000 as of June 2011 to an average of 5000 after May 2012), and the interest showed by several media outlets on the project, has shown the project to contribute a significant role in the improvement of water urban planning and building regulations.

However it must be underlined that the process of renewing Municipality rules including water aspects will require more time than expected. Although the SWM technologies and approaches proposed are of growing interest in the scientific community and are reckoned to be effective both for household [19–22] and urban contexts [23,24], the economic crisis is progressively reducing the activities of Municipalities in the environmental sector and—according to the experience of WATACLIC project—water now has a very low ranking in the interest of public administrations.

8.3.2 WATER TARIFFS AND OTHER ECONOMIC INSTRUMENTS

Water tariffs and the cost of water services have been key topics of public debate in Italy during the past years (the national referendum held in June 2011 established that water management services could not be operated by private companies). On the other hand, the uncertainty of the general legal framework and the unclear position of Water Authorities (ATO) has very often brought the discussion, during the water and money events, to embrace more general issues, rather than concentrating on tariff schemes and other economic instruments able to discourage high domestic consumption, guarantee infrastructure development and maintenance [25–27], and stimulate new technologies (rain water harvesting, greywater re-use).

In May 2012 the Italian Energy Authority, after the Law n. 214/2011 [28] assigned to the same Authority competencies on Water Services Regulation, started a public consultation on a new national water tariff scheme. In the meantime, while general public opinion is still very much worried about the possible growth of water tariffs, the environmental movement requests full application of the "polluter pays" principle, clearly saying that the huge investments in the water sector needed to fulfill the requirements of the Directive 2000/60, have to be paid by water users.

Thus, the WATACLIC team is confident that in a reasonable time (hopefully before new general elections in April 2013) the objective of WATACLIC (to adopt tariff schemes aimed at discouraging unwise use of water) will be reached at a national scale, by a new national tariff scheme; WATACLIC will have certainly contributed to such a result, as well as enhancing and stimulating the debate on these issues among relevant stakeholders.

More difficult will be the adoption of economic tools to stimulate new technologies. A proposal circulated during WATACLIC campaigns to include some water technologies (rain water harvesting, greywater re-use) among the building restoration solutions that receive fiscal incentives to promote energy efficiency, raised interest by Environmental NGOs but has not yet achieved public debate.

8.3.3 EFFICIENCY OF THE WATER SUPPLY SYSTEM

It is probably the most sensitive topic for Italian public opinion, and there is a general agreement that something has to be done to reduce water losses in a large part of the distribution networks, particularly in the south of Italy. The WATACLIC campaign water and energy concerned very technical aspects and was targeted at a very technical audience: nevertheless participation was very high. The proposed technical solutions to improve water and energy efficiency of distribution networks are in the WATACLIC database, downloadable from the website, and they will be disseminated far beyond the project lifespan as their efficacy is well documented [29,30]. Several Water Utilities that have been involved in the organization of the WATACLIC campaign (Hera, ACEA, Iren, AMAP, Abbanoa) are planning interventions to reduce water losses and the WATACLIC partner responsible for the campaign (University of Bologna), is already providing scientific advice to some of them. Thus, it is reasonable to forecast a significantly positive impact of the WATACLIC project on the topic. It is more difficult to quantify the expected reduction of losses, as well as to predict a plausible timetable: the possibility to act, in fact, depends on the availability of financial resources, which is linked to the new tariff scheme and to other financial aspects that are still on the table.

To further increase the impact of the project on this topic, and also to press for political commitments from the water utilities, Federutility (the Italian association of all public companies managing water in the country) will be involved as partner in the organization of the WATACLIC final conference and, after the project end, as co-promoter of the national annual communication campaign (water "wise" use national day).

8.3.4 RAISING AWARENESS OF FINAL USERS AND OF PROFESSIONAL PLUMBERS

The campaigns water and citizens and water and innovation—the first one targeted at several actors organizing awareness raising campaigns for the general public, the second one targeted to professional plumbers to inform them about sustainable water management technologies—are the campaigns that achieved the worst results, in terms of participation at the events.

The WATACLIC team, however, is confident that the objective "to adopt more effective awareness raising campaigns directed to the general public" will be attained, at least partially. The topic of "how to communicate water saving concepts to citizens" needs to be re-considered, once the new tariffing scheme has been adopted. Communication campaigns, in fact, could be much more effective. Additionally, a clear "price signal" on the value of water needs to be given.

The lack of interest by plumbers and by the sector industries is probably the most problematic issue. Project targets—apparently quite easy to meet and to be involved in—were not fully reached, even though the structure of the events was simplified and adapted to allow more replication of the events and a wider participation. The objective "to improve knowledge and awareness of plumber professional organization concerning water saving techniques" has therefore only partially been achieved.

It appears to be very clear that the "environmental awareness" of the industrial sector will not contribute very much to disseminate "sustainable" technologies, if the market (specifically households and the building industry) does not ask for them. The campaigns presented very interesting technologies and products already available on the Italian market (e.g., very efficient toilets using less than five liters for a complete flush), but apparently water efficiency is not an important criterion used to select bathroom and toilet equipment by final users.

Besides legally binding building regulations and price signals, a wider policy is needed to inform citizens about the water consumption "performance" of toilet equipment and household appliances; something similar to what already exists for energy consumption.

8.4 CONCLUSIONS

In Italy, compared to other environmental issues, water saving and sustainable urban water management are only of low interest among the general public and specific audiences, such as public administrations and the relevant industrial sectors. The domestic and urban water issue is perceived as a problem only in the case of a poor distribution service and, even among experts, there is a very little awareness about the important logical links related to water, such as:

- Water abstraction → decrease water flow of rivers and groundwater → increase in pollution risk;
- Water use → increase with dilution of wastewater → higher costs and lower treatment efficiency;
- Urban design → rainwater management → water pollution and flood risk.

However it has been demonstrated that when the problems related to water as a scarcity or as a flood risk became relevant and the people in charge of their management perceived them as such, then the activities and campaigns that they put into practice can be very effective (see Table 6).

Water tariffing should be correctly used to assure the "full sustainability" (environmental, social and financial) of the water management system. A "demand side management" instrument, tariffing system should discourage water abstraction: including water losses in the distribution process and, through "price signaling", excessive consumption by final users. Fulfilling the "full cost recovery" principle, water tariffs should guarantee the financial sustainability of water service operators and of their investments. Last but not least, tariffs should take into consideration the low-income population, avoiding water costs becoming unaffordable. Carefully designed, economic instruments could also play a role to reduce the hydrological impact of soil sealing and urban pollution load (wastewater and diffuse pollution) to water bodies.

Another key action is to improve knowledge transfer by introducing new concepts and approaches on water management among high-level teaching institutions (high schools and universities), which are already showing a high interest.

In order to speed the process up, the elaboration of national prescriptive guidelines on "water correct" urban planning would be helpful, together with design and building regulations as well as a training course for public officers involved in urban planning.

Table 6. A few examples of sustainable water management programs at international level.

City	Problem targeted	Actions adopted	Results	Source
Zaragoza, Spain	Water scarcity, particularly a drought in the early 1990s	-Reduction of network losses; -Introduction of regulations for urban and buildings development aiming at reducing final consumption; -Communication campaigns addressed at the general public -Water Rates (surcharge on water use); - Leak Prevention and Detection (minimize leakage within individual residences as well as the water distribution system itself);	Decline in per capita domestic water consumption from 136 liters 2000 to 105 in 2009	[31]
Fukuoka, Japan	Frequent and severe droughts resulting in major water shortages for the city	-Residential Indoor Use (Water- saving devices have been installed; -Landscaping/Outdoor Use (The city also encourages the collection and re-use of rainwater for outdoor watering needs to reduce the usage of potable water). -To reduce the impact of soil sealing; - To design the wastewater network (with special reference to combined sewer overflows and extended retention basins); - To favor rainwater retention.	Data have shown that water savings from Fukuoka's water distribution regulation system amount to approximately 5 million liters per day and that Fukuoka City consumes about 20% less water than other comparably sized cities	[32]
Bruxelles, Belgium	Flood risks		New building regulations such as rainwater collection measures and green roof for new settlements have been established	[33]

In order to increase the awareness about the water issue, institutions, public bodies, and NGOs have to promote and organize a national long term educational, cultural and information program, targeted at all categories of stakeholders. Broad communication campaigns, coordinated at national level and implemented by regional and local partners, are needed.

When the previous actions have been accomplished, the rest will follow: water management companies will invest to improve their systems, local authorities will update their urban planning and building regulations and—together with NGOs—they will organize effective information campaigns, final users will look for more efficient technologies and the market (plumbing and building operators and sanitation industry) will answer positively.

REFERENCES

1. EU (European Union). Establishing a framework for Community action in the field of water policy. In Water Framework Directive 2000/60. Official Journal of the European Union: Brussels, Belgium, 2000. Available online: http://eur-lex.europa.eu/LexUriServ/LexUriServ.do?uri= OJ:L:2000:327:0001:0072:en:PDF (accessed on 11 December 2012).
2. ISPRA (Istituto Superiore per la Protezione e la Ricerca Ambientale). Annuario Dati Ambientali 2011 (in Italian); ISPRA: Roma, Italy, 2012. Available online: http://annuario.isprambiente.it (accessed on 27 September 2012).
3. IPCC (Intergovernmental Panel on Climate Change). Fresh water resources and their management. In Contribution of Working Group II to the Fourth Assessment Report of the Intergovernmental Panel on Climate Chang; Parry, M.L., Canziani, O.F., Palutikof, J.P., van der Linden, P.J., Hanson C.E., Eds.; Cambridge University Press: Cambridge, UK, 2007; Chapter 3. Available online: http://www.ipcc.ch/publications_and_data/ar4/wg2/en/ch3.html (accessed on 27 September 2012).
4. EU. Adapting to Climate Change: Towards a European Framework for Action; Technical Paper for Commission of the European Communities: Brussels, Belgium, 2009. Available online: http://ec.europa.eu/clima/policies/adaptation/documentation_en.htm (accessed on 27 September 2012).
5. EEA (European Environmental Agency). Towards Efficient Use of Water Resources in Europe; Report n.1/2012; EEA: Copenhagen, Denmark, 2012. Available online: http://www.eea.europa.eu/ publications/towards-efficient-use-of-water (accessed on 27 September 2012).
6. EEA. Use of Freshwater Resources (CSI 018); EEA: Copenhagen, Denmark, 2010. Available online: http://www.eea.europa.eu/data-and-maps/indicators/use-of-freshwater-resources/use-of- freshwater-resources-assessment-2 (accessed on 27 September 2012).

7. UTILITATIS 2010—Studio ed Elaborazione di un Quadro Operativo per l'impianto Gestionale dei Servizi Pubblici Locali (in Italian); Report Commissioned by the Presidenza del Consiglio dei Ministri, Dipartimento Affari Regionali: Roma, Italy, 2010.
8. Zetland, D. Global Water Tariffs Continue Upward Trend. GWI (Global Water Intelligence), September 2011; Volume 12, Issue 9. Available online: http://www.globalwaterintel.com/ archive/12/9/market-profile/global-water-tariffs-continue-upward-trend.html (accessed on 27 September 2012).
9. ISTAT.IT. (Istituto Nazionale di Statistica Online Databases). Available online: http://www.istat.it/it/prodotti/banche-dati (accessed on 27 September 2012).
10. EEA. Water in the City. Available online: http://www.eea.europa.eu/articles/water-in-the-city (accessed on 27 September 2012).
11. Larsen, T.; Gujer, W. The concept of sustainable urban water management. Water Sci. Technol. 1997, 35, 3–10.
12. Li, Z.; Boyle, F.; Reynolds, A. Rainwater harvesting and greywater treatment systems for domestic application in Ireland. Desalination 2010, 260, 1–8.
13. Fangyue, L.; Wichmanna, K.; Otterpohl, R. Review of the technological approaches for grey water treatment and reuses. Sci. Total Environ. 2009, 407, 3439–3449.
14. Otterpohl, R.; Buzie, C. Wastewater: Reuse-oriented wastewater systems—Low- and high-tech approaches for urban areas. In Waste, a Handbook for Management, 1st ed.; Letcher, T., Vallero, D., Eds.; Academic Press: Boston, MA, USA, 2011; Chapter 9, pp. 127–136.
15. Masi, F. Water reuse and resources recovery: The role of constructed wetlands in the Ecosan approach. Desalination 2009, 246, 27–34.
16. Araujo, L.S.; Ramos, H.; Coelho, S.T. Pressure control for leakage minimisation in water distribution systems management. Water Resour. Manag. 2006, 20, 133–149.
17. Mutikanga, H.E.; Vairavamoorthy, K.; Sharma, S.K.; Akita, C.S. Operational tools for decision support in leakage control. Water Pract. Technol. 2011, 6, DOI:10.2166/wpt.2011.057.
18. Charlesworth, S.M.; Harker, E.; Rickard, S. Sustainable Drainage Systems (SuDS): A soft option for hard drainage questions? Geography 2003, 88, 99–107.
19. Domènech, L.; Saurí, D. A comparative appraisal of the use of rainwater harvesting in single and multi-family buildings of the Metropolitan Area of Barcelona (Spain): Social experience, drinking water savings and economic costs. J. Clean. Prod. 2011, 19, 598–608.
20. Fewkes, A. The use of rainwater for WC flushing: the field testing of a collection system. Build. Environ. 1999, 34, 765–772.
21. Dixon, A.; Butler, D.; Fewkes, A. Water saving potential of domestic water reuse systems using greywater and rainwater in combination. Water Sci. Technol. 1999, 39, 25–32.
22. Liu, B.; Ping, Y. Water saving retrofitting and its comprehensive evaluation of existing residential buildings. Energy Procedia 2012, 14, 1780–1785.
23. Otterpohl, R.; Grottker, M.; Lange, J. Sustainable water and waste management in urban areas. Water Sci. Technol. 1997, 35, 121–133.
24. Charlesworth, S. A review of the adaptation and mitigation of global climate change using sustainable drainage in cities. J. Water Clim. Chang. 2010, 1, 165–180.

25. Massarutto, A. Water pricing and full cost recovery of water services: Economic incentive or instrument of public finance? Water Policy 2007, 9, 591–613.
26. Massarutto, A.; Paccagnan, V.; Linares, E. Private management and public finance in the Italian water industry: A marriage of convenience? Water Resour. Res. 2008, 44, W12425:1–W12425:17.
27. OECD (The Organisation for Economic Co-operation and Development). Pricing Water Resources and Water and Sanitation Services; OECD Publishing: Paris, France, 2010.
28. Save Italy Act; Law No. 214/2011; Gazzetta Ufficiale: Rome, Italy, 2011.
29. Bolognesi, A.; Bragalli, C.; Marchi, A.; Artina, S. Genetic heritage evolution by stochastic transmission in the optimal design of water distribution networks. Adv. Eng. Softw. 2010, 41, 792–801.
30. Cabrera, E.; Pardo, M.A.; Cobacho, R.; Cabrera, E. Energy audit of water networks. J. Water Resour. Plan. Manag. 2010, 136, 669–677.
31. Smits, S.; Bueno Bernal, V.; Celma, J. Zaragoza: Taking Pride in Integrated Water Management in the City; IRC WASH Library: The Hague, The Netherlands, 2010. Available online: http://www.irc.nl/page/62396 (accessed on 27 September 2012).
32. Kaminski, L.E. Technology and Practices outside the Great Lakes—St. Lawrence Region. Great Lakes Commission: Ann Arbor, MI, USA, 2004. Available online: http://www.glc.org/wateruse/conservation/pdf/BestTechnologiesReport.pdf (accessed on 27 September 2012).
33. Bruxelles Environnement, l'administration de l'environnement et de l'énergie de la Région de Bruxelles-Capitale (In French). Available online: http://www.bruxellesenvironnement.be/Templates/Particuliers/informer.aspx?id=3906 (accessed on 27 September 2012).

CHAPTER 9

Full-Scale Implementation of a Vertical Membrane Bioreactor for Simultaneous Removal of Organic Matter and Nutrients from Municipal Wastewater

SO-RYONG CHAE, JIN-HO CHUNG, YONG-ROK HEO, SEOK-TAE KANG, SANG-MIN LEE, AND HANG-SIK SHIN

9.1 INTRODUCTION

Eutrophication is a key driver causing a number of pressing environmental problems including reductions in light penetration and increases in harmful algal blooms. It is known as that wastewater is an important point source for N and P loading in many aquatic environments [1]. In nutrient-sensitive estuaries, municipal and industrial WWTPs are required to implement more advanced treatment methods in order to meet increasingly stringent effluent guidelines for nutrients. According to literature, biological nutrient removal (BNR) processes that incorporate coupled nitrification/denitrification have the potential to remove TN down to about 5–12 mg/L, in selected cases, down to 3 mg/L. The TN concentration in effluent is known as less than 10 mg/L at most inland municipal WWTPs [2]. However, it is thought difficult to remove bacteria effectively from the effluent of WWTPs using the conventional activated sludge (CAS) process without a disinfection facility.

One of the possible technologies to meet this need is the membrane bioreactor (MBR) [3–6]. Rejection of bacteria by microfiltration (MF) or ultrafiltration (UF) membranes has been shown to be highly effective [7,8]. Additionally, MBR provides absolute separation of hydraulic retention time (HRT) and sludge retention time (SRT), thus allowing more flexible control of the bioreactor [9]. MBR systems can offer a solution in highly populated areas, or in areas where land used to disperse bioreactor effluents can be better used for other purposes [10]. Large-scale applications of MBR in urban wastewater treatment will require new technological developments saving energy and space, and producing high quality effluents for further applications [11,12].

In these regards, we developed and optimized a novel VMBR to reduce the problems on pollutant removal from wastewater and the volume of produced sludge from a bench-scale to field-scale systems. The effects of various operating factors such as anoxic zone/oxic zone ratio, internal recycle rate, and HRT on nutrient removal were studied using a bench-scale VMBR (working volume = 32 L) fed with synthetic wastewater containing glucose as a sole carbon source [13]. Under the optimum condition (i.e., anoxic zone/oxic zone ratio = 0.6, HRT = 8 h, and internal recycle rate = 400%), the average removal efficiencies of TN and TP were 75% and 71%, respectively [13]. The effects of water temperature on nutrient removal were evaluated using a pilot-scale VMBR (working volume = 1333 L) treating municipal wastewater. During the continuous operation for one year, average removal efficiencies of TN and TP by the pilot-scale VMBR were found to be 74% and 78% at 8 h HRT, 60 d SRT and various temperatures (13–25 °C) [14,15].

In 2009, the VMBR was commercialized by Daewoo Engineering and Construction under the trade-name of Daewoo MBR (DMBR™). Currently, six full-scale plants (Q = 1100–16,000 m^3/d) are in operation in South

Korea. In this study, we report performance and stability of the full-scale plants for the long-term operation (1–5 years).

9.2 MATERIALS AND METHODS

9.2.1 OPERATING CONDITIONS OF FIELD-SCALE VMBRS

All field-scale DMBR™ systems have been identically designed and operated. The anoxic zone/oxic zone ratio and internal recycle rate were maintained at 0.6 and 4Q, respectively as reported in the previous study [13]. As shown in Figure 1, influent and mixed liquor of suspended sol-

Figure 1. Schematic diagram of a field-scale DMBRTM system.

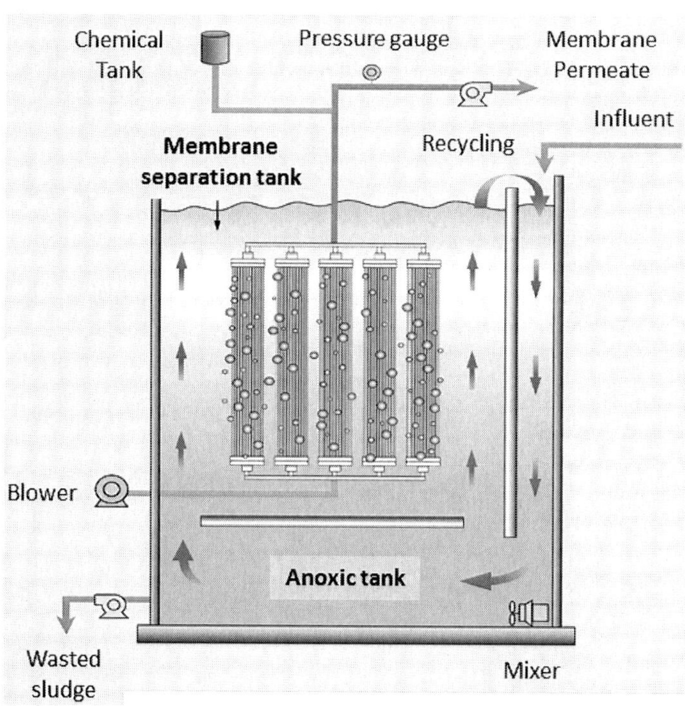

Table 1. Key information of the DMBR™ systems treating municipal wastewater larger than 1000 m^3/d.

Location in South Korea	Capacity (m^3/d)	Commission (year)	Membrane Area (m^2)	Water Temperature (°C)	HRT (h)	SRT (d)	MLSS Concentration (mg/L)
Dangjin-si (A)	3,500	2009	6,720	17.9 ± 4.5	8.3	41	9,100
Dangjin-si (B)	1,500	2009	2,560	18.1 ± 4.2	7.9	45	9,600
Gumi-si	8,000	2011	15,360	19.1 ± 3.4	8.4	40	8,500
Jecheon-si	1,100	2012	1,920	17.1 ± 5.2	9.2	37	8,900
Kwangju-si	16,000	2013	32,400	19.3 ± 3.9	8.5	38	8,500

Table 2. Characteristics of wastewater for the field-scale DMBRTM systems.

Item	Dangjin-si (A)	Dangjin-si (B)	Gumi-si	Jecheon-si	Kwangju-si
pH	7.5	7.4	7.2	7.1	7.1
BOD_5 (mg/L)	91.6	151.5	128.3	165.4	177.0
COD_{Mn} (mg/L)	90.4	97.1	96.0	53.2	89.6
SS (mg/L)	73.6	144.0	168.8	161.0	179.8
TN (mg/L)	35.3	38.5	36.3	32.0	36.6
TP (mg/L)	4.3	4.9	3.3	2.8	3.6
E. coli (cfu/100 mL)	88,660	86,443	109,747	44,101	247,795

id (MLSS) that was recycled from the oxic zone were introduced to the anoxic zone through the flow distributors. The aerobic zone is separated from the anoxic zone by a horizontal plate with a hole in the center. In the aerobic zone, disk-type diffusers were used to provide air bubbles (2800 $m^3/h = 0.42\ m^3/m^2/h$) for oxidation of organic and ammonia and to reduce membrane fouling. Final effluent was withdrawn through 0.45 μm polytetrafluoroethylene (PTFE) hollow fiber membranes (Sumitomo Electric Fine Polymer, Inc., Tokyo, Japan). A permeate pump was operated for 9 min on and 1 min off in repeating cycles. After 36 cycles, the membranes was backwashed using permeate (flow rate = 1.5Q) for 1 min. To improve removal efficiency of phosphorus, $FeCl_3$ (33%) was added into the oxic zone at 1.1 mole Fe/mole P in the feed ratio. Excess sludge was withdrawn from the anoxic zone to maintain SRT. Average HRT of the MBR systems was 8.3 h. MLSS concentration in the bioreactor varied between 8400 and 9600 mg/L depending on SRT (37–45 d) (Table 1).

Table 2 shows characteristics of municipal wastewater used for the field-scale DMBR™ systems. The COD/TN ratio and the COD/TP ratio of influent was found to be 1.8–2.6 and 19.0–29.1, respectively indicating a shortage of carbon for effective nutrient removal.

9.2.2 CHEMICAL CLEANING OF THE MEMBRANES

Two different chemical cleaning schemes were applied for mitigation of membrane fouling in the bioreactor. Firstly, an in-line cleaning is applied once a week for 30 min at 4.96 $mL/min/m^2$ using a mixture solution of NaOCl (1000 mg/L) and NaOH (100 mg/L). Secondly, an off-line cleaning was conducted if TMP reaches to 60 kPa. For this purpose, the membrane modules was removed from the bioreactor and immersed into a mixture solution of NaOCl (1000 mg/L) and NaOH (2%) for 8 h, and followed by H_2SO_4 (1%) for 8 h.

9.2.3 CHARACTERIZATION OF WASTEWATER AND MEMBRANE PERMEATE

SS and MLSS concentrations were determined by vacuum filtration of 100 mL of activated sludge through a pre-dried GF/C filter (Whatman–GE Healthcare, Pittsburgh, PA, USA) and then dried at 105 °C for 2 h. Chemical oxygen demand (COD_{Mn}), biochemical oxygen demand (BOD_5), total Kjeldahl nitrogen (TKN), NH_4–N, and TP concentrations were analyzed as described in the previous study [14]. Concentrations of various ions such as NO_2–N, NO_3–N, and ortho-P were analyzed using ion chromatography (IC) (Dionex DX-120, Sunnyvale, CA, USA) after filtering with a 0.45 μm membrane filter (ADVANTEC MFS Inc., Dublin, CA, USA). Temperature and pH were measured by temperature and pH electrodes

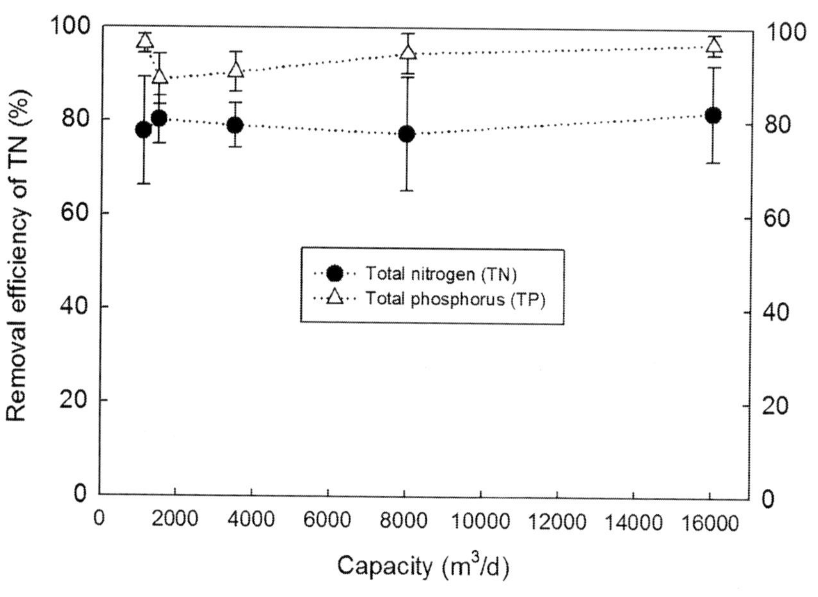

Figure 2. Average removal efficiencies of total nitrogen (TN) and total phosphorus (TP) by the full-scale DMBR™ systems (Data obtained from the full-scale DMBR™ systems for 1–5 years depending on operation period of each system).

Table 3. Performance of various submerged membrane bioreactor (MBR) systems treating municipal wastewater

MBR Type	Capacity (m3/d)	Operating Conditions	Influent Characteristics (mg/L)	TN Removal (%)	TP Removal (%)	Influent COD/TN Ratio	Reference[a]
MLE	1,375	HRT = 33 h SRT = n.a.	BOD = 114 TN = 29 TP = 3.4	78	50	3.9	[11]
MLE	2,400	HRT = 16.6 h SRT = 40 d	COD = 447 NH_4-N = 26 TP = 7.3	99	91	17.2[b]	[16]
MLE	6,520	HRT = 3.5–5 h SRT = 14–21 d	COD = 220 TN = 26 TP = 3.9	70	92	8.5	[17]
Verical MLE	1,100–16,000	HRT = 7.9–9.2 h SRT = 37–45 d	COD = 53–97 TN = 32–39 TP = 2.8–4.9	78–82	89–97[c]	1.7–2.6	This study

Notes: a BOD/TN ratio; b COD/NH_4-N ratio; c The chemical precipitation was employed using $FeCl_3$; n.a.: data was not available..

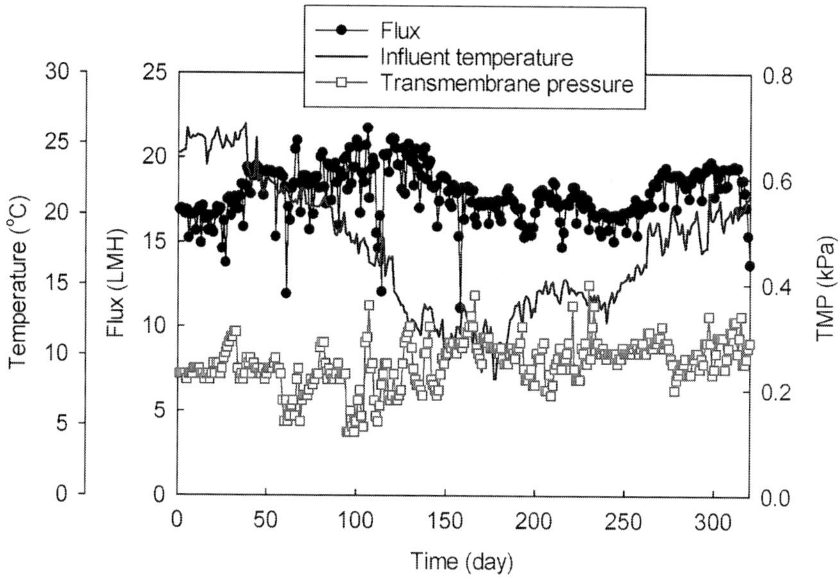

Figure 3. Progress of membrane fouling in a field-scale DMBR™ system (Dangjin-si (A), South Korea).

connected with a pH meter (Orion Model 420A, Orion Research Inc., Beverly, MS, USA). Average removal efficiency of SS, organic compounds, and nutrients by the DMBR™ systems as calculated as:

$$\text{Removal efficiency (\%)} = (1 - C_f/C_i) \times 100$$

where C_f is the final concentration in the membrane permeate and C_i is the initial concentration in the influent.

Tryptone-broth was used to enumerate *E. coli*, which was incubated at 37 °C for 24 h. Removal rejection efficiency of *E. coli* by the membrane was calculated by the following equation:

$$\text{Removal efficiency (\%)} = (1 - N_p/N_f) \times 100$$

where N_p is colony forming units (cfu) of *E. coli* per 100 mL in the membrane permeate and N_f is the cfu of *E. coli* per 100 mL in the influent.

9.3 RESULTS AND DISCUSSION

9.3.1 PERFORMANCE AND FOULING CHARACTERISTICS OF THE FULL-SCALE DMBR™ SYSTEMS

During the long-term operation of the field-scale DMBR™ systems treating municipal wastewater, it was found that organic matter (BOD_5 > 99%), particles (SS removal efficiency > 99%), and *E. coli* (>99.9%) have been effectively removed (data not shown).

Average removal efficiencies of TN and TP by the DMBR™ system were found to be 79% and 90% at 18 °C, 8.3 h HRT and 41 d SRT. Interestingly, there is no big change in removal efficiency of nutrients (TN = 78%–82% and TP = 89%–97%) regardless of the system size (Q = 1100–16,000 m^3/d) (Figure 2). Moreover, the TMP was maintained below 40 kPa with membrane permeate flux at 18 LMH more than 300 days (Figure 3).

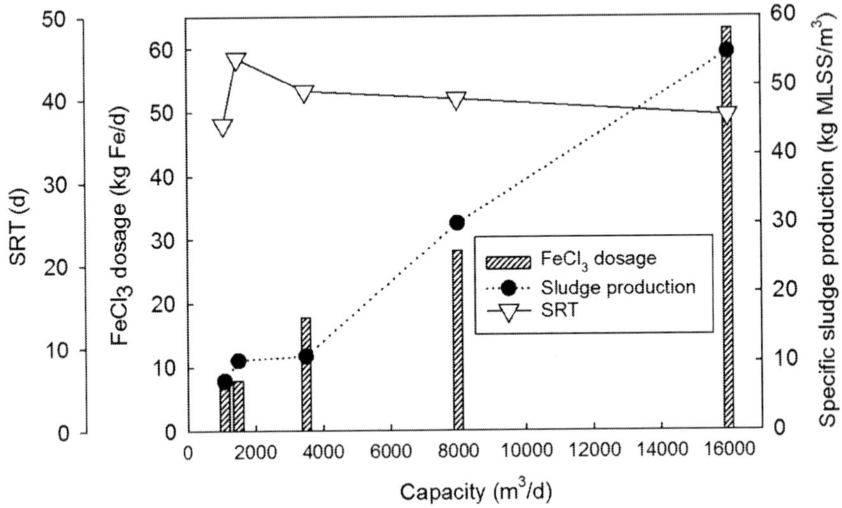

Figure 4. $FeCl_3$ dosage and sludge production from the full-scale DMBR™ systems.

Table 3 represents performance of full-scale submerged MBR systems treating municipal wastewater. System configuration of the MBR systems are similar to the Modified Ludzack-Ettinger (MLE) process (i.e., pre-denitrification followed by aerobic thank with submerged membranes). At the relatively higher COD/TN ratio (i.e., 8.5 and 17.2), the MLE-type MBRs showed good performance for both N and P removal. However, when the COD/TN ratio is low (i.e., 3.9), P removal efficiency was limited.

As shown in Table 3, the DMBR™ system showed competitive performance for nitrogen removal compared to other MBR systems even at the relatively low influent COD/TN ratio (< 3). However, P removal efficiency of the DMBR™ was below 50% (data not shown) at the low COD/TN ratio. To enhance the removal efficiency of P, $FeCl_3$ (1.1 mole Fe/mole P in the feed) was introduced into the aerobic tank resulting in 89%–97% removal of phosphorus.

9.3.2 CHEMICAL DOSAGE AND EXCESS SLUDGE PRODUCTION

Because of the unique feature of MBRs and particularly the significant decrease in membrane price, MBRs have been increasingly and widely used for wastewater treatments in the last decade [12,16,17].

However, despite these developments and applications of MBRs, energy demand together with frequent membrane cleaning remain a challenge in terms of energy consumption and optimization of MBRs [9]. Energy demand of full-scale CAS processes for municipal wastewater treatment, expressed per volume of treated wastewater was reported to be in the range of 0.1–0.6 kWh/m^3 [18]. However, energy consumption of MBRs was generally higher due to intensive membrane aeration rates required to mitigate membrane fouling and clogging than that of CAS systems. Typical energy demand values for full-scale MBR systems are reported to be in the range of 0.4–2.0 kWh/m^3 [11,18].

The energy requirement of the DMBR™ systems was in the range of 0.8–1.0 kWh/m^3 (data not shown). The specific energy consumption of the full-scale DMBR™ systems was averaged at 0.94 kWh/m^3. This is slightly higher than that of the CAS systems and some MBRs mainly due to addition of $FeCl_3$ for enhanced phosphorus removal.

On the other hand, waste activated sludge (WAS) from CAS processes is one of the most serious problems in wastewater treatment [19]. It has been known that extremely low sludge production (0.05–0.25 kg mixed liquor of volatile suspended solid (MLVSS)/kg COD) is possible for low food-to-microorganism (F/M) ratios and long SRT in MBRs [20]. In this study, $FeCl_3$ was introduced to improve P removal efficiency. However, as $FeCl_3$ dosage increased from 8 to 63 kg/d, the observed sludge yield of the full-scale DMBR™ systems was also increased from 7.2 to 54.8 kg MLSS/m^3 (or from 0.92 to 6.3 kg MLVSS/kg COD) (Figure 4).

9.4 CONCLUSIONS

Since 2009, five full-scale vertical MBR plants (Q = 1100–16,000 m^3/d) have been successfully in operation to reduce the problems concerning effective removal of nitrogen and phosphorus from municipal wastewater for water recycling. Particles (i.e., SS), organic substances (i.e., BOD_5 and COD_{Mn}), and bacteria (i.e., *E. coli*) were effectively removed (>99%) by the MBR systems. TN and TP removal efficiencies of the MBR plants were found to be 78%–82% and 89%–97%, respectively at 7.6–9.2 h HRT and 37–45 d SRT. However, the introduction of $FeCl_3$ for improvement of phosphorus removal efficiency resulted in relatively high sludge production compared to the conventional MBRs without chemical precipitation.

A stable operation was possible by applying the weekly in-line cleaning using a mixture of NaOCl and NaOH without significant increase in TMP (<40 kPa) for approximately one year with the average energy consumption of 0.94 kWh/m^3. Recycling and reuse of P removed by $FeCl_3$ will be beneficial to the MBR operation.

REFERENCES

1. Mesfioui, R.; Love, N.G.; Bronk, D.A.; Mulholland, M.R.; Hatcher, P.G. Reactivity and chemical characterization of effluent organic nitrogen from wastewater treat-

ment plants determined by fourier transform ion cyclotron resonance mass spectrometry. Water Res. 2012, 46, 622–634.
2. Grady, C.P.L., Jr.; Daigger, G.T.; Love, N.G.; Filipe, C.D.M. Biological Wastewater Treatment; IWA Publishing–CRC Press: Boca Raton, FL, USA, 2011.
3. Huang, X.; Xiao, K.; Shen, Y.X. Recent advances in membrane bioreactor technology for wastewater treatment in china. Front. Environ. Sci. Eng. China 2010, 4, 245–271.
4. Santos, A.; Judd, S. The commercial status of membrane bioreactors for municipal wastewater. Sep. Sci. Technol. 2010, 45, 850–857.
5. Le-Clech, P. Membrane bioreactors and their uses in wastewater treatments. Appl. Microbiol. Biotechnol. 2010, 88, 1253–1260.
6. Van Nieuwenhuijzen, A.F.; Evenblij, H.; Uijterlinde, C.A.; Schulting, F.L. Review on the state of science on membrane bioreactors for municipal wastewater treatment. Water Sci. Technol. 2008, 57, 979–986.
7. Tai, C.S.; Snider-Nevin, J.; Dragasevich, J.; Kempson, J. Five years operation of a decentralized membrane bioreactor package plant treating domestic wastewater. Water. Pract. Technol. 2014, 9, 206–214.
8. Arevalo, J.; Ruiz, L.M.; Parada-Albarracin, J.A.; Gonzalez-Perez, D.M.; Perez, J.; Moreno, B.; Gomez, M.A. Wastewater reuse after treatment by MBR. Microfiltration or ultrafiltration? Desalination 2012, 299, 22–27.
9. Meng, F.G.; Chae, S.R.; Drews, A.; Kraume, M.; Shin, H.S.; Yang, F.L. Recent advances in membrane bioreactors (mbrs): Membrane fouling and membrane material. Water Res. 2009, 43, 1489–1512.
10. Chae, S.-R.; Ahn, Y.; Hwang, Y.; Jang, D.; Meng, F.; Shi, J.; Lee, S.-H.; Shin, H.-S. Advanced Wastewater Treatment Using Mbrs: Nutrient Removal and Disinfection; Iwa Publishing: London, UK, 2014; pp. 137–163.
11. Itokawa, H.; Tsuji, K.; Yamashita, K.; Hashimoto, T. Design and operating experiences of full-scale municipal membrane bioreactors in Japan. Water Sci. Technol. 2014, 69, 1088–1093.
12. Meng, F.G.; Chae, S.R.; Shin, H.S.; Yang, F.L.; Zhou, Z.B. Recent advances in membrane bioreactors: Configuration development, pollutant elimination, and sludge reduction. Environ. Eng. Sci. 2012, 29, 139–160.
13. Chae, S.R.; Kang, S.T.; Watanabe, Y.; Shin, H.S. Development of an innovative vertical submerged membrane bioreactor (VSMBR) for simultaneous removal of organic matter and nutrients. Water Res. 2006, 40, 2161–2167.
14. Chae, S.R.; Shin, H.S. Characteristics of simultaneous organic and nutrient removal in a pilot-scale vertical submerged membrane bioreactor (VSMBR) treating municipal wastewater at various temperatures. Process Biochem. 2007, 42, 193–198.
15. Chae, S.R.; Shin, H.S. Effect of condensate of food waste (CFW) on nutrient removal and behaviours of intercellular materials in a vertical submerged membrane bioreactor (VSMBR). Bioresour. Technol. 2007, 98, 373–379.
16. Silva, A.F.; Carvalho, G.; Oehmen, A.; Lousada-Ferreira, M.; van Nieuwenhuijzen, A.; Reis, M.A.M.; Crespo, M.T.B. Microbial population analysis of nutrient removal-related organisms in membrane bioreactors. Appl. Microbiol. Biotechnol. 2012, 93, 2171–2180.

17. Wan, C.Y.; de Weyer, H.; Diels, L.; Thoeye, C.; Liang, J.B.; Huang, L.N. Biodiversity and population dynamics of microorganisms in a full-scale membrane bioreactor for municipal wastewater treatment. Water Res. 2011, 45, 1129–1138.
18. Krzeminski, P.; van der Graaf, J.; van Lier, J.B. Specific energy consumption of membrane bioreactor (mbr) for sewage treatment. Water Sci. Technol. 2012, 65, 380–392.
19. Guo, W.Q.; Yang, S.S.; Xiang, W.S.; Wang, X.J.; Ren, N.Q. Minimization of excess sludge production by in-situ activated sludge treatment processes—A comprehensive review. Biotechnol. Adv. 2013, 31, 1386–1396.
20. Wang, Z.W.; Yu, H.G.; Ma, J.X.; Zheng, X.; Wu, Z.C. Recent advances in membrane bio-technologies for sludge reduction and treatment. Biotechnol. Adv. 2013, 31, 1187–1199.

PART V

ENERGY CONSUMPTION

CHAPTER 10

Energy Benchmarking of Commercial Buildings: A Low-Cost Pathway toward Urban Sustainability

MATT COX, MARILYN A. BROWN, AND XIAOJING SUN

10.1 INTRODUCTION

Commercial buildings accounted for nearly one-fifth of the energy consumed in the US in 2010, and their portion of the nation's energy budget is expected to increase to 21% by 2035 (EIA 2011a). Commercial buildings dominate the urban landscape, and their energy requirements contribute to urban air quality and heat island effects. As a result, innovative policies that promote energy-efficient commercial buildings are critical to sustainable development. We focus here on the use of energy benchmarking to inform building owners and tenants about poor-performing buildings and subsystems and to enable high-performing buildings to achieve greater occupancy rates, rents, and property values. We estimate the possible impacts of a national policy mandating the energy benchmarking of US commercial buildings, emphasizing the benefits to sustainable urban development.

The commercial building sector suffers from three main information failures. First, there is the problem of information asymmetry: building owners and managers know more about the energy performance and efficiency of their buildings than prospective buyers and tenants. Analogous to the case of 'lemons' in the used car market as described by Akerlof (1970), this can lead to inefficient transactions. Second, there are principal–agent problems in the sector, which occur when one party (the agent) makes decisions in a market and a different party (the principal) bears the consequences. This issue was found by Prindle (2007) to be significant and widespread in many end-use energy markets in both the US and other countries. In many commercial buildings, architects, engineers, and builders select equipment, duct systems, windows, and lighting for future building occupants. Similarly, landlords often purchase and maintain appliances and equipment for tenants who pay the energy bill, providing little incentive for the landlord to invest in efficient equipment (Brown 2001). Third, a decades-long research effort has identified discount rates related to equipment purchases that are far higher than theoretically anticipated, resulting in fewer purchases of high-efficiency equipment (Frederick et al 2002, Train 1985).

This analysis focuses on giving building owners in the country access to baseline information on their building's energy consumption ('benchmarking'), which is currently unavailable or underutilized in most parts of the US. This could be accomplished by requiring utilities to submit energy data in a standard format to a widely used database, such as Portfolio Manager [1], which currently maintains information on hundreds of thousands of buildings in the US, provided by building owners and managers. Using existing software packages, meter data from utilities and building owners could be combined to provide a 'virtual building meter', allowing for building-wide assessments [2]. The data would then be available to the building owner and the utility and maintained by the Environmental Protection Agency (EPA).

According to a report sponsored by the US Green Building Council and others (Carbonell et al 2010), the EPA may have the authority to require utilities to submit building energy data under section 114 of the Clean Air

Act. This utility data must be connected to individual buildings to be useful in providing building owners with baseline energy performance information. A uniform national building identification system, similar to the VIN system for cars, could facilitate this connection regardless of where a building is located, how it is used, or whether it has multiple street addresses—all currently issues for energy benchmarking.

The benchmarking approach assessed here involves two features.

- Utilities are required to submit whole building aggregated energy consumption data for all tenants to the EPA Portfolio Manager.
- A national registry of commercial buildings, with each building receiving a unique building identification (BID) number is developed.

If implemented, better building energy data would become available to owners, tenants, and utilities. In turn, benchmarking efforts could be accelerated; demand side management programs could become more feasible; municipal governments would have a uniform system for building codes and mandated disclosure reporting; and the federal government would gain valuable data to inform the ENERGY STAR® building certification standards and the commercial building energy consumption survey. The real estate sector would be able to provide better information to clients, and energy performance could be better incorporated into property assessments.

10.2 BACKGROUND

Benchmarking creates an energy consumption baseline for a specific building. If benchmarking is completed for a large set of buildings and stored in a shared database, comparisons become possible. Benchmarking also helps to set priorities for limited staff time and capital. EPA and the American Council for an Energy-Efficient Economy (ACEEE) both suggest that savings up to 10% can be made at little or no cost to building owners, savings which are frequently overlooked (Dunn 2011, Nadel 2011).

The federal government benchmarks its buildings as a result of Section 432 of the Energy Independence and Security Act of 2007. However, policy experience with benchmarking in the US is largely tied to mandated disclosure policies at the state and local level (figure 1). Most of these policies emphasize the residential sector or are under consideration, but six cities and two states (California and Washington) have adopted mandated disclosure, which necessitates benchmarking of commercial buildings. Every existing American program, including an international effort between the US and Canada, uses Portfolio Manager as the benchmarking tool (EPA 2011). As of 2012, Portfolio Manager includes data on the performance of more than 300 000 buildings in the US, providing normalized building scores that qualify buildings for ENERGY STAR certification and help achieve LEED certification.

The Institute for Market Transformation (IMT) summarized recent experiences of nine current US programs (Burr et al 2011). As a result of program reviews and in-depth stakeholder discussions, a series of best practices were recommended for benchmarking, the main one being to follow EPA guidelines surrounding the use of the Portfolio Manager. This recommendation enables jurisdictions to avoid debates over building use and building type classifications, but there are other benefits as well, including easy integration of building data into the Portfolio Manager format.

10.2.1 RESULTS FROM IMPLEMENTING GOVERNMENTS [3]

While Europe has used mandated disclosure and benchmarking programs for many years, the US is just beginning to implement these programs. Currently, the governments of New York City, Seattle, Washington, DC, Philadelphia, and Austin, Texas are taking leadership roles (Keicher et al 2012, Burr et al 2011). Results have begun to be released, notably in New York City, where 2010 and 2011 data have been reported for over 2000 buildings. The 2010 report suggested that if the bottom half of large commercial buildings could be brought to just the median level of energy performance, energy consumption and greenhouse gases from this building class would fall by 18% and 20%, respectively (City of New York 2012a). The summary of the 2011 release suggests that such an effort would reduce total citywide greenhouse gases by 9% (City of New York 2012b).

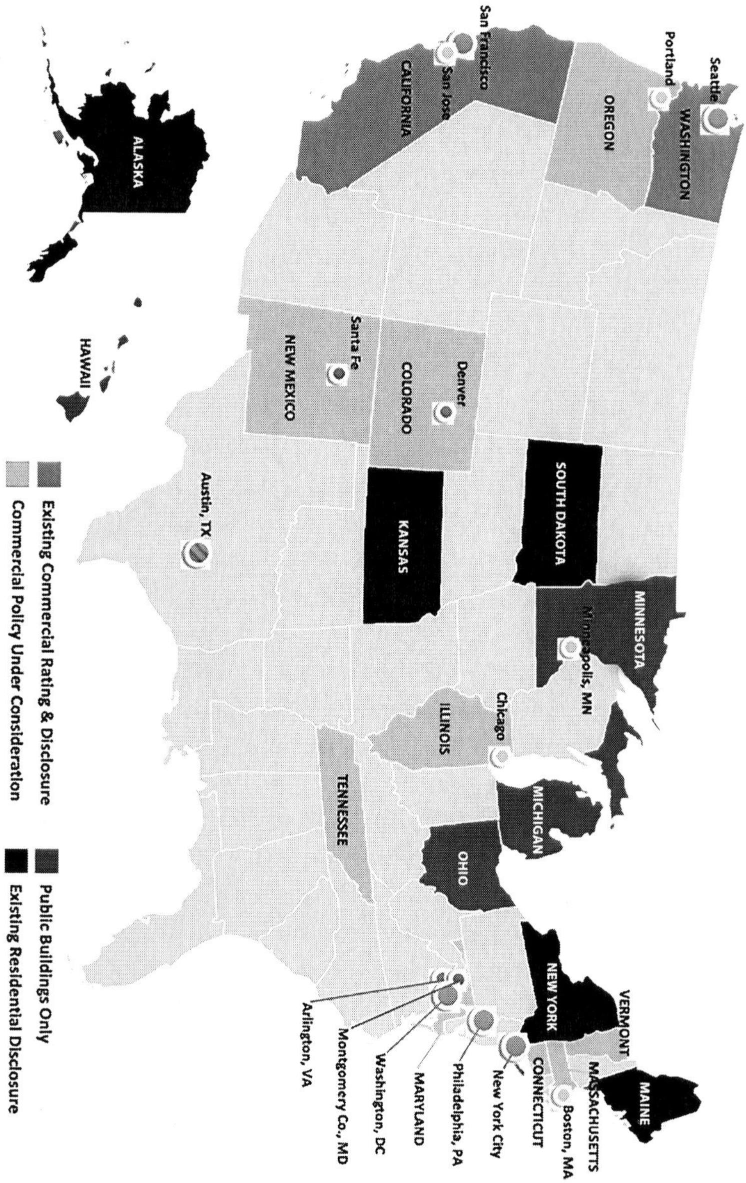

Figure 1. Mandated disclosure and benchmarking efforts in the US. Reproduced with permission from Burr (2012).

Table 1. Main conclusions from program managers.

Core lessons from program managers	Key areas for assistance
• Portfolio Manager and the SEED database are great tools • Programs are reducing information gaps • Implementation is more difficult than anticipated • Building aggregation capacity is crucial	• Clarifying leadership roles at the federal level • Workforce certification programs • Defining confidential data • Funding or rules for utilities to aggregate building data and facilitate release and access

Interviews with key program managers from leading cities discovered consistent findings that can be informative for policymakers (table 1).

First, Portfolio Manager has found broad acceptance as the principal benchmarking tool. The time-series and cross-sectional comparison capabilities of the tool make it extremely attractive. The Standard Energy Efficiency Data Platform [4] that DOE provides has also been well receive because it helps the local governments share best practices. However, the dual-agency approach has led to confusion about federal roles, and some cities have suggested that clarifying leadership positions would be helpful.

Second, all program managers interviewed believe a large information gap related to building energy consumption existed in their jurisdictions prior to the benchmarking and mandated disclosure laws. While benchmarking efforts have assisted in reducing this gap by informing building owners about total building performance, the gap remains.

Third, tenant authorization is required for building owners to access energy consumption data in many jurisdictions. Rules and support for utilities to facilitate easy access and release of aggregated building data are particularly important. One manager stated that if he were starting over, aggregated building data rules would be the first thing instituted.

Fourth, every program experienced delays in implementation, largely due to the economic downturn in 2008. Frequently, timelines had to be amended after the program began in earnest. Lastly, a commonly noted issue is the lack of a qualified workforce—certification programs for contractors are strongly desired. Benchmarking and mandated disclosure efforts have the potential to create and expand markets for energy contractors, and some means to differentiate between contractors would reduce other information barriers for building owners.

10.2.2 POLICY RATIONALE

'Policy actions. . . could, in principle, correct for the excessive present-mindedness of ordinary people' (Solow 1991).

Benchmarking has the potential to reduce information asymmetries in the marketplace and to lower the discount rates used by consumers in the sector. A few scholars question the extent and evidence of such problems (Alcott and Greenstone 2012, Gillingham et al 2009, Jaffe and Stavins 1994). This skepticism seems to stem from the information assumptions of neoclassical economics. Policy tools based on such theory are unable to modify discount rates and provide no policy relevant advice for information-based gaps (Stern 1986). In contrast, empirical research has found that information can modify discount rates in use; providing information may address a barrier to the deployment of energy-efficient technologies that other approaches cannot.

Theoretically, one way discount rates are determined is by combining the market interest rate with a time preference premium and some level of uncertainty or risk; with efficient capital markets, discount rates should converge with interest rates (Fuchs 1982). Hausman theorized that rational actors would equate the potential stream of energy savings from more efficient technologies with the monetary savings from buying less-expensive equipment. His findings on implicit discount rates, however, did not match the theory; for efficient air conditioners, consumers used discount rates that were much higher than the market interest rate. 'Other factors such as uncertainty and the possibility of technological change do not seem sufficient to explain the high discount rate which we found' (Hausman 1979). Later research would find many instances where empirically observed discount rates deviated from theoretical predictions, finding that future gains receive higher discounting than future losses (Thaler 1981), that smaller anticipated results (either positive or negative) receive higher discount rates than larger anticipated results (Benzion et al 1989), and that consumers prefer improving sequences of outcomes (Frederick and Loewenstein 2002, Varey and Kahneman 1992). Furthermore, Sultan and Winer (1993) found no evidence of consumers using market-based discount rates across a number of appliances.

Research specific to equipment-purchasing decisions found numerous discount rates in use across the population. These discount rates vary over time and appliances (Train 1985, Koomey 1990). Frederick and Loewenstein (2002), in a review of the theoretical and empirical history of discount rates, found the following.

The implicit discount rate was 17–20% for air conditioners (Hausman 1979); 102% for gas water heaters, 138% for freezers, 243% for electric water heaters (Ruderman et al 1987); and from 45% to 300% for refrigerators, depending on assumptions made about the cost of electricity (Gately 1980).

Disparate findings in discount rates across the population pose theoretical difficulties, but open the door for different policy approaches and rationales. Tools in regulatory, financial, and information areas may help to address discount rate issues: for example, equipment standards and subsidies can result in choices that approximate the effect of lowering discount rates by eliminating low-efficiency choices and reducing first cost, respectively. However, information-based policies have the unique ability to modify the discount rate in use. Studies have found that providing information can reduce discount rates anywhere from 3% to 22% (Coller and Williams 1999, Goett 1983). Coller and Williams suggest that information about energy consumption will result in a 5% decline in discount rates for energy decisions made by the median population. Depending on the discount rate in use, an adjustment of this size could dramatically impact equipment decisions.

In the commercial sector, numerous studies (Christmas 2011, Campbell 2011, Miller et al 2008, Jackson 2009, Das et al 2011) show higher occupancy rates, higher rents, and higher property values for high-efficiency buildings. Benchmarking could increase the market demand for these buildings. Portfolio Manager itself has the potential to address some information gaps through its use of time-series data and cross-sectional comparisons. This may lead to more energy-efficient technology choices, reduced uncertainty in maintenance costs, lower fuel costs, and ease the attainment of building certifications like ENERGY STAR. The ties between Portfolio Manager and ENERGY STAR certification also reduce transaction costs for renters desiring high-performance space. This could reduce the size of the principal–agent problem by creating market and social pressure for building owners to consider energy in purchasing decisions, particularly when combined with mandated disclosure.

Recent studies show that benchmarking spurs energy efficiency investments (NMR Group, Inc. with Optimal Energy, Inc. 2012), one of the fastest, direct, and cost-effective means of reducing greenhouse gas emissions (Ciochetti and McGowan 2010). To the extent that benchmarking limits the emission of greenhouse gases, it helps to correct this negative externality and mitigates the threat posed by climate change. In essence, benchmarking has the potential to be a step toward better consumer choices without resorting to pricing instruments or regulation. In this way, it is a policy tool complementary to economically efficient approaches such as carbon pricing policies, guiding behavioral changes by energy managers and users. With the commercial sector representing 19% of US CO_2 emissions (over 3% of global emissions), and that percentage expected to grow (DOE 2012), managing the emissions of the sector is critical to 'preventing dangerous interference with the climate system' (UNFCCC 1992).

10.3 METHODOLOGY

Technological selection in many modeling efforts is based on a series of economic considerations such as first costs and discount rates. The impact on energy consumption is not insignificant, as the efficiency of technologies available for meeting the same demand for energy services in the marketplace is quite varied. For modeling projections, technological forecasting, technological assessment and progress, as well as social factors that influence the adoption of technologies, are critical (Coates et al 2001). Such forecasting and modeling efforts face long odds of accurately projecting future outcomes, but can be useful in providing estimates as well as informing policy debates (Silberglitt et al 2003). Furthermore, many models also struggle with simulating macroeconomic spillover effects, where actions taken in one sector of the economy change conditions and thus alter decisions in other sectors of the economy.

Our analysis of benchmarking in the commercial sector utilizes the Georgia Tech version of the Energy Information Administration's (EIA) 2011 National Energy Modeling System (GT-NEMS) (a detailed description of the NEMS commercial module, which was modified for this study, can be found in the Commercial Demand Module of the National Energy Modeling System: Model Documentation (EIA 2011b)). GT-NEMS contains a technology menu and forecast developed from manufacturer surveys of anticipated technological performance for several hundred types of equipment. GT-NEMS also has the capacity to simulate macroeconomic spillover effects. When selecting a technology in the commercial sector to meet a demand for energy services, GT-NEMS uses a combination of discount rates and the rate for US government ten-year Treasury notes to calculate consumer 'hurdle rates' used in evaluating equipment-purchasing decisions. While the macroeconomic module of GT-NEMS determines the rate for ten-year Treasury notes endogenously, the discount rates are exogenous. Modifying these inputs is the primary means of estimating the impact of benchmarking for the commercial sector in this analysis. This is done in two steps: first, by updating the discount rates to reflect a broader selection of the literature; and second, by adjusting the updated discount rates to account for the effects of a national benchmarking policy.

The GT-NEMS inputs for discount rates are separated by end use, including space heating, space cooling, ventilation, lighting, water heating, cooking, and refrigeration, divided into seven population segments for each end use. Each population segment is capable of using a different discount rate with regard to the end use in question each year. In the Annual Energy Outlook 2011 (EIA 2011a) reference case, these discount rates are quite high; for example, more than half of the consumer choices in lighting and space heating use discount rates greater than 100%, and less than 3% of the population uses discount rates under 15% (EIA 2011b).

Such high discount rates are not reflected by the bulk of the existing research. This problem has been recognized for some time in energy forecasting models (Decanio and Laitner 1997). An extensive literature review spanning four decades uncovered more than two-dozen studies estimating implicit discount rates for commercial consumers across the GT-NEMS series of appliances. The mean discount rates in this literature ranged from 17% (space heating and space cooling both) to 63% (refrigerators). The simulation and econometrics to analyze risk (SIMETAR) [5] tool was used to develop continuous probability distribution functions for each end use. GRKS distributions were used for space cooling, lighting, cooking, and water heating. SIMETAR matched Weibull distributions as a better fit for space heating and refrigeration. Ventilation was the sole end use to have no specific studies; the space heating distribution was used to represent it (see supplementary material, available at stacks. iop.org/ERL/8/035018/mmedia, for full details of the discount rates and distributions used in the modeling).

Ideally, the continuous functions would be used to model the distribution of discount rates across the population. However, GT-NEMS is not suited for this due to the segmented approach previously described. Therefore, the probability density functions were divided into seven segments of equal area for each end use. The median value of these seven segments generates the updated discount rates scenario (UDR). To estimate the impact of benchmarking, two scenarios were modeled. In the Benchmarking 5% scenario, the findings of Coller and Williams (1999) were applied, meaning the median value declined by five percentage points. The quotient of this 'benchmarked' median discount rate and the updated median discount rate was calculated and used as an adjustment factor to the other six population segment medians. In this way, the findings of Coller and Williams are carried throughout the consumer population, since each population segment reduces by the same proportion as the median. Given the uncertainty in the estimates of information-based discount rate modifications and the wide range of reported implicit discount rates (Train 1985), we also produce the Benchmarking 10% scenario, which follows the same method but applies a 10% reduction to the median discount rate from the UDR scenario.

GT-NEMS adds the rate of ten-year Treasury notes to these values, which vary by year according to macroeconomic conditions. The reference case Treasury note rates were subtracted from the updated discount rates so that the final hurdle rate calculated by GT-NEMS are consistent with the values suggested by the literature. These modifications generate the main policy cases: 'Benchmarking 5%' and 'Benchmarking 10%'. All policy scenarios begin implementation in 2015.

A number of sensitivities were also modeled, where benchmarking pushes R&D forward, bringing new, highly efficient technologies to the marketplace. This sensitivity (referred to as 'Benchmarking +') utilizes the EIA High Tech technology suite for the commercial sector where 40 new high-efficiency technologies are introduced (EIA 2011a), and is consistent with the 'announcement effect', which describes the phenomenon that firms and customers adjust their behavior in the interim between the announcement of a regulation and its implementation. However, it needs to be acknowledged that there is still a gap between the High Tech assumptions and state-of-the-art technologies that are currently available in the market place. This analysis would be more thorough if GT-NEMS could account for the latest developments in technology innovation and deployment. Furthermore, the benchmarking policy combined with whole building design practices that consider the design, operations, and maintenance of buildings could lead to greater impacts. For example, GT-NEMS accounts for the operations and maintenance costs of equipment; however, the provision of energy information through a benchmarking policy could lead building owners to improve overarching operations and maintenance regimes (such as shell characteristics), which could be an unaccounted-for benefit of this policy approach.

To give a sense of the uncertainty in the analysis, two alternative scenarios are included that bound the potential benefits of modifying the discount rates of consumers. Energy expenditures are expected to severely impact the total benefits of the policy. The high benefits case reflects a future where EPA regulations make it more expensive to keep using coal for base-load power, resulting in higher electricity prices. As a result, consumers will demand more efficient technologies, and manufacturers will deliver these. To model this, we utilize the assumptions of the AEO 2011 High Coal Cost side case and the High Tech side case technology menu. The low benefits case reflects a case where there are diminished prices for coal, perhaps from reduced demand due to cheap natural gas. At the same time, we expand estimates of supply for shale gas, resulting in lower gas prices than in the GT-NEMS reference solution. This scenario uses the reference case technology suite. A description of the side cases can be found in AEO 2011 (EIA 2011a).

The macroeconomic module of GT-NEMS handles some other uncertainties, like growth in population and commercial building stocks. An increase in population and growth in the commercial sector are anticipated by the model; for example, commercial floor space is projected to increase by 32.7% between 2012 and 2035. However, none of the benchmarking policy scenarios modeled in this analysis have any discernible impact on population or commercial building stock growth rates. Faster increases in either of these variables would increase energy demand and related emissions.

10.4 RESULTS

10.4.1 TECHNOLOGY SHIFTS

In both 2020 and 2035, the greatest savings are from natural gas space heating, followed by ventilation. Electric space heating experiences an increase in consumption after 2025, following the adoption of more heat pumps in those years. Excluding ventilation, the average saving for an end use is 1% in 2020 and 1.2% in 2035 in the Benchmarking 10% scenario.

Both benchmarking scenarios result in a series of technology shifts across the major end uses. For space heating, GT-NEMS projects a fuel shift from natural gas to electric technologies. Benchmarking 5% mostly shows service demand shifting within each fuel type, but also a trade of 4 TBtu in service demand between natural gas space heating and electric space heating in 2020. By 2035, this service demand trading increases to 18 TBtus, accounted for by a shift toward electric heat pumps. Benchmarking 10% follows a similar trajectory; in 2020, the single most significant change in service demand is a move from typical natural gas furnaces to high-efficiency natural gas furnaces. However, by 2035, about 30 TBtus in service demand for natural gas heating are shifted to air-source heat pumps, representing a change in the fuels and technologies selected by consumers to meet space heating demand. This technology shift is partially responsible for greater natural gas savings than electricity. However, the energy price context is constantly evolving. GT-NEMS projects increasing natural gas prices, but a prolonged presence of cheap natural gas may drive the private sector to develop more and better natural gas end-use technologies, which could affect commercial sector technology choices.

10.4.2 REDUCED ENERGY CONSUMPTION AND EXPENDITURES

The benchmarking policy scenarios modeled in this study all target the seven major equipment classes that account for approximately 45% of the energy used by commercial buildings: space heating, space cooling, ventilation, lighting, water heating, cooking, and refrigeration. The impact can be seen in figure 2. The updated discount rate reduces projected energy consumption by 4.0% in 2020 and 8.7% in 2035, for these seven energy end uses. This finding suggests that the EIA reference case overestimates future US energy consumption by underestimating future investments in energy-efficient building equipment. Analysis of forecasts from the 1980s relative to actual US energy use indicates that this overestimation bias is long-standing (Laitner 2009).

Benchmarking 5% shows savings of 1.3% in 2020 (150 TBtu) and 2.2% (260 TBtu) in 2035 when compared to the UDR case. Benchmarking 10% projections are slightly larger at 1.4% (160 TBtu) in 2020 and 2.4% (270 TBtu) in 2035. In 2020, the high benefits case produces a 3.7% decline in energy consumption from the UDR case, rising to 10% in 2035.

Benchmarking reduces energy consumption without reducing the commercial sector's growing spatial footprint. As a result, energy intensity, measured in Btu ft^{-2}, declines, as does the nation's energy intensity as a whole. In 2020, benchmarking results in a 1% improvement in energy intensity, relative to the UDR case.

Benchmarking 10% shows reduced energy demand over the modeling horizon; both natural gas and electricity consumption is down an average of 1.6% compared to the UDR case. The result is a reduction in the average price for natural gas of 0.3%. When Benchmarking 5% is compared to the UDR case, natural gas and electricity consumption decline by an average of 2.2% and 1.4%, respectively, with a corresponding 0.2% and 0.3%

average reduction in price for each fuel. Rebound effects, where lower levels of energy consumption reduce prices and thus increase energy consumption, contribute to limiting energy savings in the modeled scenarios (Sorrell et al 2009).

Decreased demand combined with declining energy prices result in a reduction in energy expenditures by the owners of commercial buildings. Compared with the UDR case, Benchmarking 10% expenditures drop by 0.7% in 2020, saving $1.2 billion; in 2035, expenditures drop 1.1%, saving $2.4 billion. On average, annual energy expenditures drop by 0.7%, valued at $1.4 billion. These savings cumulatively total $13 billion through 2035, and $16 billion over the lifetime of the installed equipment (at a 7% discount rate). In Benchmarking 5%, 2020 expenditures drop 0.8%, worth $1.5 billion; 2035 expenditures drop 0.9% and are worth $1.9 billion. Savings through 2035 have a net present value of $11 billion, increasing to $13 billion over the lifetime of the equipment (also at a 7% discount rate). While the savings appear modest compared to some other energy efficiency programs (Brown et al 2013, Gillingham et al 2006), we have shown that these differences change technology choices in the commercial sector, and we will show that they are still meaningful on the supply side and with respect to environmental benefits.

Several NEMS features may have restricted the energy-saving potential. First, NEMS models the discount rates used by commercial customers for only seven equipment classes. Office equipment and miscellaneous end uses [6] are modeled through a different, simplified fashion with negligible efficiency improvements. In reality, a benchmarking policy could reduce energy consumption of all end uses, which means the consumption reduction presented in figure 2 is at the low-end of the saving potential. In addition, the technology choice decision rule used in NEMS presents a barrier to higher energy savings. According to the model, when it comes to end-use equipment retrofit or placement, consumers have a certain freedom in choosing technologies, but the majority of them are limited to use either a later version of the same technology or at least remain in the same fuel type. At a minimum, this restricts fuel switching in the sector and could potentially stop consumers from choosing economically feasible high-efficiency technology and dampen the energy savings. Previous studies of energy economic models (including NEMS) have found evidence

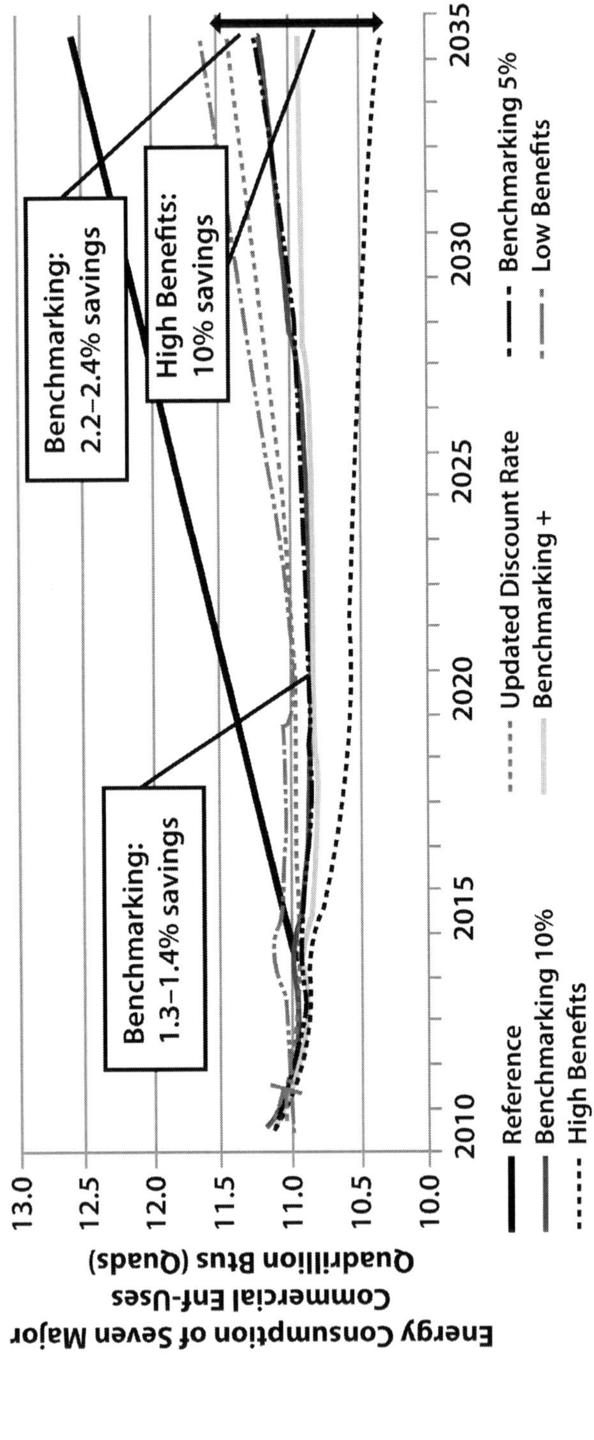

Figure 2. Major end-use commercial sector energy consumption.

that these models tend to reinforce the status quo, underestimate innovation (in both policy and technology), and miss market potential, issues that may explain some of the modest savings potential for benchmarking projected by GT-NEMS (Laitner et al 2003, Laitner 2009).

10.4.3 COST EFFECTIVENESS

While the benchmarking policy option is modeled as ceasing in 2035, the benefits of the policy would extend into the future due to the lifetime of energy-saving technologies installed as a result of the policy. Energy-efficient technologies have varying lifetimes (for example, chillers and boilers last longer than natural gas water heaters) [7]. This analysis assumes that energy savings degrade at 5% annually (Brown et al 1996). Therefore, technologies installed in 2035 provide the greatest savings in that year, with a linear decline in savings out to 2055, when energy savings are no longer expected. The same rationale is applied to emissions benefits.

Aside from the private sector benefits from reduced energy expenditures, there are social benefits from fewer pollutant emissions. Our analysis includes criteria pollutant (SO_2, NO_x, and $PM_{2.5}$ and PM_{10}) benefits and CO_2 benefits. Changing the regulatory framework for these pollutants and other changes (lower prices or innovations, for example) that result in dramatic departures from projected means of meeting energy demand would lead to different estimates of the costs and benefits associated with these pollutants.

Criteria pollutant benefits are calculated based on values from the National Research Council (2010), and take into account public health effects, damage to crops and timber, buildings, and recreation. Such damage tends to vary substantially depending on meteorological conditions, proximity of populations to emitters, and the sources and means of electricity generation (Fann and Wesson 2011). The National Research Council estimates exclude damage from mercury pollution, climate change, ecosystem impacts, and other areas where damage is difficult to monetize. Even with this incompleteness, damage from coal power plants is estimated to exceed $62 billion annually, and recent analysis suggests that the damage from coal power plants exceeds the value added to the economy (Muller et al 2011). The national average values provided for electricity generation and on-site use of energy sources are used to analyze the emissions benefits of benchmarking.

Carbon dioxide emissions are outputs of GT-NEMS and are the result of fuels used for energy on-site and in the electricity sector. The economic value of reductions in CO_2 is estimated by multiplying the annual decrement in emissions by the 'social cost of carbon' (SCC). In this analysis, the central values of the US Government Interagency Working Group on the Social Cost of Carbon (EPA 2010) are used, ranging from \$25 per metric ton of CO_2 in 2015 to \$47 per metric ton of CO_2 in 2050 (in 2009-\$).

Benchmarking policies improve the ability of the market to operate effectively and take advantage of low-cost energy-saving opportunities. As a result, the damage from pollutants declines, representing significant public benefits over the duration of the policy timeline analyzed here. However, the two benchmarking scenarios strongly diverge on the emissions benefits. This is due to discontinuities in demand side choices that impact supply side decisions. For example, GT-NEMS projects a temporary increase in the use of coal for electric generation in the East North Central census division in the Benchmarking 5% scenario. This is largely due to national reductions in electricity consumption, reducing the price of coal and increasing the attractiveness of coal-fired electric generation in the decade post-policy initiation. The Benchmarking 10% scenario produces similar reductions in both natural gas and electricity, creating price effects that favor natural gas generation in the electric sector, particularly from combined heat and power. The result is that increased coal consumption and the related increase in emissions projected under Benchmarking 5% are avoided by Benchmarking 10%. The supply side is behaving very differently in these two cases. This non-linearity accentuates the value of a general equilibrium framework, because such uncertainties, tipping points, and supply–demand interplays would not otherwise be visible.

When compared to the UDR case, the cumulative value of avoided criteria pollutant emissions is estimated at \$1.4–3.4 billion in 2020, growing to \$3.0–8.2 billion in 2035 (ranges reported for Benchmarking 5% and Benchmarking 10% using a 3% discount rate). Including CO_2 benefits, the net present value of these emissions reductions would be \$3.9–10.5 billion through 2035 with the potential to grow to more than $18 billion over the lifetime of equipment installed under the policy.

To put these emissions reductions in perspective, we estimated the scale of installed capacity required to achieve the same level of CO_2 mitigation from nuclear power and solar photovoltaics, as other carbon-free electricity sources. In 2020, the Benchmarking 5% and 10% projections show reductions of 4–22 million metric tons (MMT) CO_2 relative to the UDR case. Based on the average carbon intensity of grid-supplied electricity projected by GT-NEMS, achieving these carbon reductions requires replacing 7.2–39.7 TWh of electricity generation in 2020 with carbon-free generation. Nuclear power typically has a much higher capacity factor than solar; for the purposes of this comparison, we assume an 89% capacity factor. In 2020, this would require 925 MW–5.1 GW of nuclear power. Assuming a capacity factor of 17% for solar photovoltaics, achieving the same carbon savings would require 4.8–26.6 GW of solar capacity.

While the reductions in CO_2 are significant, this result adds to a growing body of literature that is skeptical of technological innovation and behavioral change as sufficient to address the threat of climate change—regulatory and taxation approaches may well prove necessary (van den Bergh 2013). The US government has established goals for energy reductions in the commercial sector (the Better Buildings Initiative, aiming for a 20% reduction from projected 2020 energy consumption in commercial buildings) and greenhouse gas reductions for the entire economy (a 17% reduction in CO_2 from 2005 levels, established at the Copenhagen climate negotiations in 2009). Benchmarking policies can assist but many other initiatives will be necessary to achieve these goals.

Turning to costs associated with benchmarking, buildings with multiple tenants will require aggregation services in order to determine the energy footprint of an entire building. We call these compliance costs. These costs were determined using the 2003 Commercial Building Energy Consumption Survey (CBECS) data (EIA 2007), which provides the number of multi-tenant buildings with electric and natural gas services. The average square footage of a multi-tenant building from CBECS is used in conjunction with GT-NEMS projections of commercial floor space to produce estimates of the number of multi-tenant buildings that will exist between 2004 and 2035. Burr (2012) estimates that existing laws will require 60 000 buildings to undergo benchmarking regardless of this policy option, so these are subtracted from the total. It is assumed that compliance costs will be the same for each building, following the Consolidated Edison model in New York City, and is set at $102.50 (2011-$) for electricity and natural gas. Consolidated Edison provides both gas and electric data for $102.50, a value that was calculated based on anticipated labor costs to collect and aggregate data and approved by the New York State Public Service Commission (Consolidated Edison Company 2010). We model that a building needing aggregation for both fuels would incur costs of $205, based on the assumption that gas and electric services may not be provided by the same utility in every jurisdiction, making our estimate of cost higher than would likely be the case. The end result is an initial cost of $141 million (2009-$) in 2015. Costs for new buildings after 2015 are also included, ranging from $2.7 million in 2016 to $3.2 million in 2035 (2009-$).

These costs are modeled as public costs due to concerns about distributional impacts and policy viability. If these costs were directed to utilities, opposition would likely grow substantially. The costs of accounting upgrades and software development are probably minor, but the cost of benchmarking every building would not be. If costs were directed toward building owners, they would be incentivized to avoid complying. As the purpose of the policy is to identify and benchmark the energy consumption of as many buildings as possible in the US, that outcome would not complement the policy goals. Therefore, it is recommended that the federal government finance the compliance costs, distributing funding through special grants to utilities at levels determined by the proposed BID system. Such an approach would alleviate increased utility opposition and foster a cooperative environment.

Lastly, the costs associated with equipment are handled by GT-NEMS and determined from model outputs. Costs for installation, operations, maintenance, and eventual removal at the end of equipment life are estimated, showing reductions in cost under both benchmarking scenarios due to declining service demands. Investment costs for the major end uses are derived from the technology-specific details about energy service demand, technology cost per unit of energy service demand, and annual usage characteristics [8].

Table 2. Benefit–cost analysis of commercial sector benchmarking[a] (billion 2009-$)

	Cumulative social benefits					Cumulative social costs		Cost–benefit analysis
Year	Value of avoided CO_2	Energy expenditure savings	Value of avoided criteria pollutants	Lower equipment outlays	Total benefits	Compliance costs	Total costs	Net social benefits
2020	6.3–2.8	−0.4–0.1	1.4–3.4	6.4–5.4	13.7–11.7	0.1	0.1	
2035	28.3–22.0	0.6–1.6	3.1–7.3	18.0–21.7	50.0–52.6	0.1	0.1	
Total impact[b]	39.7–31.7	0.9–2.3	3.0–8.2	18.0–21.7	61.5–63.8	0.1	0.1	61.4–63.7

[a] Present value of costs and benefits were analyzed using a 3% discount rate. Values reported in table 2 are the Benchmarking 5% value followed by the Benchmarking 10% value.

[b] The total impact accounts for the energy savings and its related benefits occurring throughout the lifetime of the commercial equipment, assuming an average lifetime of 20 years..

One shortcoming of this modeling approach is the weak linkage between demand for new equipment in one sector and the energy consumption related to its production in the industrial sector. The implication for our study is that the embedded emissions and energy consumption of producing equipment used in retrofits (i.e. replacing existing equipment before the end of equipment life with a more efficient unit) is not observable. The Commercial Building Energy Consumption Survey suggests that these types of retrofits affect less than 0.8% of buildings annually (EIA 2007), and a much smaller percentage of overall equipment purchases. Benchmarking is anticipated to increase the rate of retrofits. While GT-NEMS determines retrofit decisions, it does not separately report them, eliminating our ability to estimate 'missing' energy consumption or emissions. However, for equipment purchased in new buildings or to replace expired equipment, the model is capable of more accurately assessing the associated industrial energy consumption and emissions.

Having tallied the benefits and costs of benchmarking to both the private and public sector, it is worthwhile to see how these compare from a societal perspective. In the first five years of the policy, compliance costs and the increases in criteria pollutant emissions are significant costs, but the commercial sector is showing net benefits of $11.6–13.6 billion compared to the UDR case. By 2035, cumulative energy savings, combined with the benefits of reduced emissions, exceed cumulative equipment and compliance costs by more than $40 billion. Once all new equipment has been retired, net benefits have grown to $61–64 billion using a 3% discount rate (table 2).

As is always the case with a benefit–cost analysis, there are costs and benefits that we are unable to capture, so it is crucial to recognize this effort as an incomplete best guess (Krutilla 1967). For example, the benefits of improved asset values for building owners and local governments, as well as numerous environmental benefits, are lacking from this analysis. A major benefit of benchmarking is the reduced transaction costs necessary to learn about building energy performance. Reducing these transaction costs is likely to be a large part of the policy rationale behind pursuing a policy like benchmarking, but methods to estimate the value of reduced transaction costs are currently lacking. Mandated disclosure laws would further reduce these costs.

Policymakers at all levels of government should consider that benchmarking could enable other policies, providing synergistic effects. For example, an analysis of the impact of a national commercial building code in the US projected 2035 energy savings of 0.94 Quads compared to the AEO 2011 reference case [9]. The difference in commercial sector energy consumption between the reference case projection and the benchmarking scenarios for the same year is 1.33–1.35 Quads. If these policies were purely additive, then the expected result of having both policies in effect would be a reduction of 2.27–2.29 Quads. However, when modeled together, a slight synergy was shown in the model outputs, with reductions totaling 2.30–2.35 Quads. While these are small savings, benchmarking's benefits could be expanded if matched wisely with other energy policies. Local policymakers have matched benchmarking with mandated disclosure laws and with financing programs, which may be synergistic pairings.

GT-NEMS shows that the benefits of this policy option are also sensitive to substitution effects and cross price elasticities with respect to fuel choices in the utility sector. One sensitivity scenario we ran cut shale gas reserves by 50% from the reference case. The result was a dramatic expansion in the use of coal for electricity generation in the Midwestern region of the USA. In this scenario, energy prices and expenditures increased, and emissions benefits were largely eliminated. If the assumptions within the model about fuel price elasticities in the utility sector are correct, fuel switching may severely reduce the benefits of this policy option. The assumptions in this sensitivity case may be extreme, but they highlight an additional concern for policymakers—to ensure maximum benefits from benchmarking and other similar policy options, it may be necessary to take complementary actions that decrease the incentives to use coal. Such an action would prevent backsliding in emissions benefits.

Our review of the literature surrounding discount rates and the obvious impact of the updated discount rates scenario relative to the AEO 2011 reference case suggests that the Energy Information Administration should adjust the discount rates used in the NEMS model. Doing so would create a clearly measurable change in the technologies selected to meet energy demand in the commercial sector, impacting energy consumption, prices, and pollutant emissions projections from the model used to analyze national energy policy proposals.

Urban sustainability could be improved by this policy. Currently, the US lack data on the number and type of commercial buildings and their associated energy consumption in metropolitan statistical areas (MSAs)—hence our proposal of creating the BID system. However, GT-NEMS shows a 0.997 correlation between GDP and commercial floor space. 89% of 2010 US GDP occurred within US MSAs (US BEA 2010). Assuming GDP is a useful proxy for commercial sector benefits within MSAs, we would expect to see 89% of the benefits of this policy flow to MSAs. This would result in $55–57 billion in net societal benefits.

10.5 SUMMARY

Inefficient buildings contribute to sustainability problems in urban areas. Many improvements in commercial building energy efficiency could be driven by requiring utilities to submit building energy data to a uniform database accessible to building owners and tenants. Numerous other non-monetized advantages would also present themselves as a result of the proposed BID system.

With benchmarking, the market can see more clearly the advantage of superior energy performance, potentially spurring an end-user-driven shift. Building owners would have motivation to seek highly energy-efficient tenants, perhaps even incentivizing these tenants. Private organizations or government could grant recognition of quality energy management to specific tenants, further reducing transaction costs between tenants and building owners. This could enable market-based rewards for good energy practices by tenants, perhaps something similar to an ENERGY STAR program for tenants that allowed them to signal quality practices.

The impact of benchmarking shows a reduction in energy consumption of 160–180 TBtus over the UDR case in 2035, with nearly 90% of these savings benefiting metropolitan areas. It is estimated that the benefits of a benchmarking policy outweigh the costs, both to the private sector and society broadly. The net benefits of the policy are likely underestimated, due to the inability to fully monetize all potential benefit streams. For example, we do not incorporate the benefits of building envelope improvements such as low-emissivity windows and better insulation, and we do not monetize the full suite of environmental benefits from lower electricity consumption such as the health benefits of avoided mercury pollution and the ecosystem benefits of reduced coal mining. Overcoming some of the information barriers in the sector looks to be a worthy investment, mostly on the basis of the potential for energy savings. Opposition to benchmarking is likely to be grounded in concerns over principal–agent issues, tenant privacy, incurred costs (depending on policy design and implementation), and fear of the impact on the value of poor-performing buildings. Clarity from the federal government in policy design could substantially help cities address some of this opposition and improve the functionality of the marketplace.

ENDNOTES

1. EPA Portfolio Manager www.energystar.gov/index.cfm?c=evaluate performance.bus portfoliomanager.
2. Certain utilities, like Consolidated Edison and Austin Energy, have developed meter aggregating tools to collect whole-building energy consumption data.
3. Program managers from New York City, Seattle, Austin, Washington, DC, and DOE's Building Technology Program were interviewed.
4. DOE Standard Energy Efficiency Data Platform: www1.eere.energy.gov/ buildings/commercial/seed platform.html.
5. SIMETAR: www.njf.nu/filebank/files/20070101$194034$fil$T0GT zTCK EgEZBdBS1jll.pdf.
6. Examples of miscellaneous uses includes service station equipment, automated teller machines, telecommunications equipment, and medical equipment.
7. See tables 5.3.9, 5.6.9, and 5.7.15 in the DOE Buildings Energy Data Book http://buildingsdatabook.eren.doe.gov/.
8. See section 4.7 and appendix A for more details: www.spp.gatech.edu/ faculty/workingpapers/wp69.pdf.
9. www.spp.gatech.edu/faculty/workingpapers/wp71.pdf.

REFERENCES

1. Akerlof G A 1970 The market for 'lemons': quality uncertainty and the market mechanism Q. J. Econ. 84 488–500
2. Alcott H and Greenstone M 2012 Is there an energy efficiency gap? J. Econ. Perspect. 26 3–28
3. Benzion U, Rapoport A and Yagil J 1989 Discount rates inferred from decisions: an experimental study Manag. Sci. 35 270–84 Brown M A 2001 Market failures and barriers as a basis for clean energy policies Energy Policy 29 1197–207
4. Brown M A, Baer P, Cox M and Kim Y J 2013 Evaluating the risks of alternative energy policies: a case study of industrial energy efficiency Energ. Effic. at press (doi:10.1007/s12053-013- 9196-8)
5. Brown M A, Wolfe A, Bordner R, Goett A, Kreitler V and Moe R 1996 Persistence of DSM Impacts: Methods, Applications, and Selected Findings EPRI TR-106193 (Oak Ridge, TN: Oak Ridge National Laboratory and Synergic Resources Corporation for the Department of Energy and Electric Power Research Institute)
6. Burr A C 2012 Benchmarking and Disclosure: State and Local Policy Design Guide and Sample Policy Language (Washington, DC: State and Local Energy Efficiency Action Network) (www1.eere.energy.gov/seeaction/pdfs/ commercialbuildings benchmarking policy.pdf)
7. Burr A C, Keicher C and Leipziger D 2011 Building Energy Transparency: A Framework for Implementing US Commercial Energy Rating and Disclosure Policy (Washington, DC: Institute for Market Transformation) (www.imt.org/uploads/ resources/files/IMT-Building Energy Transparency Report. pdf)
8. Campbell I A 2011 Tapping into a trillion dollar industry: how to increase energy efficiency financing by 2015 The 5th Annual Energy Efficiency Finance Forum (Washington, DC: American Council for an Energy-Efficient Economy) (www.aceee.org/ files/pdf/conferences/eeff/2011/2011presentations.pdf)
9. Carbonell T, Fidler S and Douglas S 2010 Using Executive Authority to Achieve Greener Buildings: A Guide for Policymakers to Enhance Sustainability and Efficiency in Multifamily Housing and Commercial Buildings (Washington, DC: Van Ness Feldman, PC) (www.vnf.com/assets/ attachments/USGBC%20report%20 4-29-10.pdf)
10. Christmas J 2011 Financing energy efficiency in the commercial building sector: is there hope post-PACE? The 5th Annual Energy Efficiency Finance Forum (Washington, DC: American Council for an Energy-Efficient Economy) (www.aceee.org/ files/pdf/conferences/eeff/2011/2011presentations.pdf)
11. Ciochetti B and McGowan M 2010 Energy efficiency improvements: do they pay? J. Sustain. Real Estate 2 305–33
12. City of New York 2012a plaNYC: New York City Local Law 84 Benchmarking Report
13. City of New York 2012b LL84 Benchmarking Data Disclosure Coates V, Farooque M, Klavans R, Lapid K, Linstone H A,
14. Pistorius C and Porter A L 2001 On the future of technological forecasting Technol. Forecast. Soc. Change 67 1–17 Consolidated Edison Company 2010 Re: Case 09-E-0428 Con Edison's Electric Rate Case, New York

15. Coller M and Williams M 1999 Eliciting individual discount rates Exp. Econ. 127 107–27
16. Das P, Tidwell A and Ziobrowski A 2011 Dynamics of green rentals over market cycles: evidence from commercial office properties in San Francisco and Washington DC J. Sustain. Real Estate 3 1–22
17. Decanio S J and Laitner J A 1997 Modeling technological change in energy demand forecasting a generalized approach Energy Demand Forecast. 263 249–63
18. Department of Energy (DOE) 2012 Buildings Energy Data Book (http://buildingsdatabook.eren.doe.gov/)
19. Dunn C 2011 Benchmarking in Portfolio Manager for State and Local Governments and EECBG Recipients (https://energystar. webex.com/energystar/lsr.php?AT=pb&SP=TC& rID=48542237&act=pb&rKey=d4c4f84f6ed9952c)
20. Energy Information Administration (EIA) 2007 Commercial Building Energy Consumption Survey (www.eia.gov/ consumption/commercial/)
21. Energy Information Administration (EIA) 2011a Annual Energy Outlook 2011 DOE/EIA-0383(2011) (www.eia.gov/forecasts/ aeo/pdf/0383(2011).pdf)
22. Energy Information Administration (EIA) 2011b Commercial Demand Module of the National Energy Modeling System: Model Documentation 2011 (www.eia.gov/ FTPROOT/ modeldoc/m066(2011).pdf)
23. Fann N and Wesson K 2011 Estimating PM2.5 and Ozone-Related Health Impacts at the Urban Scale (www.epa.gov/airquality/ benmap/docs/ISEE BenMAP.pdf)
24. Frederick S and Loewenstein G 2002 The Psychology of Sequence Preferences (Cambridge, MA: MIT)
25. Frederick S, Loewenstein G and O'Donoghue T 2002 Time discounting and preference: a critical time review J. Econ. Lit. 40 351–401
26. Fuchs V 1982 Time preferences and health: an exploratory study Economic Aspects of Health ed V Fuchs (Chicago: University of Chicago Press) pp 93–120
27. Gately D 1980 Individual discount rates and the purchase and utilization of energy-using durables: comment Bell J. Econ. 11 373–4
28. Gillingham K, Newell R and Palmer K 2006 Energy efficiency policies: a retrospective examination Annu. Rev. Environ. Resour. 31 161–92
29. Gillingham K, Newell R and Palmer K 2009 Energy efficiency economics and policy Resources for the Future (http://rff.org/ rff/documents/RFF-DP-09-13.pdf)
30. Goett A 1983 Household appliance choice: revision of REEPS behavioral models Final Report for Research Project 1918-1 (Palo Alto, CA: Electric Power Research Institute)
31. Hausman J 1979 Individual discount rates and the purchase and utilization of energy-using durables Bell J. Econ. 10 33–54
32. Jackson J 2009 How risky are sustainable real estate projects? An evaluation of LEED and ENERGY STAR development options J. Sustain. Real Estate 1 91–106
33. Jaffe A and Stavins R 1994 The energy paradox and the diffusion of conservation technology Resour. Energy Econom. 16 91–112
34. Keicher C, Antonoff J, Hooper B, Beber H, Pogue D and Cook L 2012 Lessons learned from the implementation of rating and disclosure policies in US cities Proc. Conf. 2012 ACEEE Summer Study on Energy Efficiency in Buildings pp 151–62
35. Krutilla J 1967 Conservation reconsidered Am. Econ. Rev. 57 777–86

36. Koomey J 1990 Energy efficiency in new office buildings: an investigation of market failures and corrective policies PhD Dissertation University of California, Berkeley, CA
37. Laitner J A 2009 The Positive Economics of Climate Change Policies: What the Historical Evidence Can Tell Us (Washington, DC: American Council for an Energy-Efficient Economy)
38. Laitner J A, DeCanio S J, Koomey J G and Sanstad A H 2003 Room for improvement: increasing the value of energy modeling for policy analysis Util. Policy 11 87–94
39. Miller N, Spivey J and Florance A 2008 Does Green Pay Off? (Working Paper) (San Diego, CA: University of San Diego)
40. Muller N, Mendelsohn R and Nordhaus W 2011 Environmental accounting for pollution in the United States economy Am. Econ. Rev. 101 1649–75
41. Nadel S 2011 Buildings energy efficiency policy: a brief history
42. Presentation made at Federal Policy Options Workshop for Accelerating Energy Efficiency in Commercial Buildings (www.ornl.gov/sci/ees/etsd/btric/ccpt comm.shtml)
43. National Research Council (NRC) 2010 Hidden Costs of Energy: Unpriced Consequences of Energy Production and Use (Washington, DC: The National Academies Press)
44. NMR Group, Inc., with Optimal Energy, Inc. 2012 Statewide Benchmarking Process Evaluation Volume 1: Report (www. calmac.org/publications/Statewide Benchmarking Process Evaluation Report CPU0055.pdf)
45. Prindle B 2007 Quantifying the Effects of Market Failures in the End-Use of Energy (Paris: International Energy Agency) (http://s3.amazonaws.com/zanran storage/www.aceee.org/ ContentPages/4790329.pdf)
46. Ruderman H, Levine M D and McMahon J E 1987 The behavior of the market for energy efficiency in residential appliances including heating and cooling equipment Energy J. 8 101–24
47. Silberglitt R, Hove A and Shulman P 2003 Analysis of US energy scenarios Technol. Forecast. Soc. Change 70 297–315
48. Solow R 1991 Sustainability: an economist's perspective Presented as the Eighteenth J. Seward Johnson Lecture at Woods Hole Oceanographic Institute (Woods Hole, MA)
49. Sorrell S, Dimitropoulos J and Sommerville M 2009 Empirical estimates of the direct rebound effect: a review Energy Policy 37 1356–71
50. Stern P C 1986 Blind spots in policy analysis: what economics doesn't say about energy use Policy Anal. 5 200–27
51. Sultan F and Winer R 1993 Time preferences for products and attributes and the adoption of technology-driven consumer durable innovations J. Econ. Psychol. 14 587–613
52. Thaler R 1981 Some empirical evidence on dynamic inconsistency Econ. Lett. 8 201–7
53. Train K 1985 Discount rates in consumers' energy-related decisions: a review of the literature Energy I 1243–53

54. United Nations Framework Convention on Climate Change (UNFCCC) 1992 http://unfccc.int/resource/docs/convkp/conveng.pdf
55. US Bureau of Economic Analysis (BEA) 2010 Gross Domestic Product by Metro Area (www.bea.gov/iTable/iTable.cfm? ReqID=70&step=1&isuri=1&acrdn=2, retrieved 31 January 2013)
56. US Environmental Protection Agency (EPA) 2010 Technical Support Document: Social Cost of Carbon for Regulatory Impact Analysis Under Executive Order 12866 (www.epa.gov/ otaq/climate/regulations/scc-tsd.pdf)
57. US Environmental Protection Agency (EPA) 2011 The Governments of United States and Canada Harmonize Approach to Save Energy in Commercial Buildings (http://yosemite.epa.gov/opa/ admpress.nsf/d0cf6618525a9efb85257359003fb69/2d85476b30cc156785257943005aafea!OpenDocument)
58. van den Bergh J C J M 2013 Environmental and climate innovation: limitations, policies and prices Technol. Forecast. Soc. Change 80 11–23
59. Varey C and Kahneman D 1992 Experiences extended across time: evaluation of moments and episodes J. Behav. Decis. Mak.5 169–85

There are several supplemental files that are not available in this version of the article. To view this additional information, please use the citation on the first page of this chapter.

CHAPTER 11

Energy Pattern Analysis of a Wastewater Treatment Plant

PRATIMA SINGH, CYNTHIA CARLIELL-MARQUET, AND ARUN KANSAL

11.1 INTRODUCTION

The growing scarcity of water has increased the dependency of urban water system on energy, both for conveyance and treatment. Access to energy can become a hindrance to the sustainable urban cities causing both shortage of water resources and water pollution. In addition, with growing climate concerns, energy saving, energy efficiency and energy substitution have become a common development principle all over the world (Friedrich et al. 2008). In this light, urban sanitation is a sector that can have substantial energy burden and can become important for power demand estimations in the coming years. This aspect is more important in developing countries where a huge gap exists between wastewater generation and treatment. In coming years, a large number of wastewater treatment-related infrastructure projects are expected to be implemented in these countries. So far, the main factors considered in decision making of such projects are the capital and operating costs, skills required for operation, and ease of technology adaptability under local conditions. Bringing energy considerations in such decision making will offer dual advantage of energy substitution and climate change mitigation which are vital ingredients of an eco-city development program (Mahgoub et al. 2010). This aspect has an amplified relevance in countries, which are energy deficient.

In a wastewater treatment plant (WWTP), energy is used in the form of electrical, manual, chemical and petroleum. A number of studies on energy analysis of a WWTP have considered only the electrical form of energy (Devi et al. 2007a; Hellstrom 1997; Jonasson 2007; Merlin and Lissolo 2010; Middlebrooks et al. 1981). However, for exploring opportunities for energy efficiency and energy substitution, a detailed analysis of various forms of energy consumption is required. Such analysis should include share of various energy forms and energy intensity at various stages of treatment process. This paper presents an energy pattern analysis of a WWTP in an institutional area. More importantly, it demonstrates a methodological framework by which such studies can be replicated to generate data with respect to various scales of treatment and choice of treatment technology. This information will provide a sound basis for planning tools and answers to the growing debate of water-energy nexus, developing energy efficiency benchmarks for urban water sector and finding possibilities for the application of renewable energy to substitute conventional forms of energy.

11.2 DESCRIPTION OF THE STUDY SITE

The WWTP is located at TERI University, which is in an institutional area at New Delhi, India. The plant has a design capacity of 25 m^3/day and is operated for 12 h a day. The actual flow of wastewater during the study period is found to vary between 19 and 23 m^3/day. Primary sources of wastewater are: hostel having 60 residents, administrative block of the University and a kitchen. The plant has been designed for reuse of water for non-potable applications. It uses physico-chemical treatment method

Table 1 Characteristics of wastewater

Parameter	Inlet	Outlet
pH	4–9	7.5–9
COD (mg/l)	840–890	<200
SS (mg/l)	550–680	<30
BOD (mg/l)	770–755	<20
P (mg/l)	2–1.50	<0.63
S (mg/l)	3–2	<0.8
NH_4 (mg/l)	45–30	<19

using coagulants such as caustic soda and aluminium sulphate as primary treatment and filtration, adsorption and disinfection as tertiary treatment. Biological treatment based on rotating biological contactor (RBC) is used as secondary treatment. The dried sludge is used in a nearby horticulture park and the treated water for watering plants. Table 1 gives wastewater and treated water characteristics, and Fig. 1 shows the wastewater treatment scheme.

The treatment plant has the following units:

1. Sump tank: reinforced cement concrete, rectangular shape underground tank, size (3 x 2 x 2) m, having two submerged sludge pumps (one as standby) each of 0.75 kW motor for feeding raw wastewater.
2. PST: rectangular shaped MS tank, size (3 x 1 x 2.25) m, fitted with one SS turbine plate stirrer with 0.19 kW motor.
3. Chemical dosing tanks: three tanks each of 100 l capacity with total 3 dosing pumps (1 pump as standby) having 0.19 kW motor.
4. RBC: tank of size (2 x 0.8 x 0.8) m; discs fitted with a worm gear motor of 0.19 kW.
5. Disinfectant tanks: two tanks each of 100 l capacity with total 3 dosing pumps (1 pump as standby) having 0.19 kW motor.

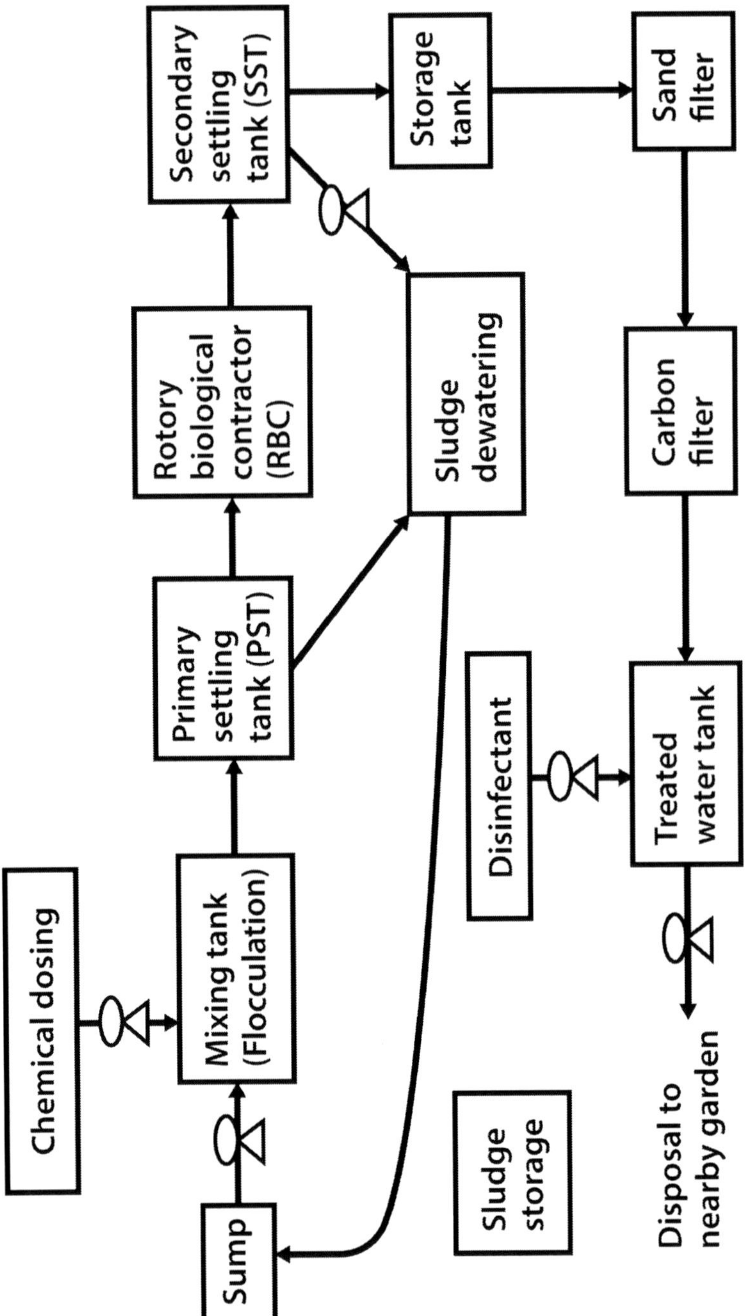

Figure 1. Process flow diagram of the WWTP

6. SST: tank of size (3 x 1 x 2.25) m, fitted with SS turbine plate stirrer 0.19 kW motor and single stage monoblock recirculation pump of 0.38 kW.
7. Sand filter and carbon filter: 200 l capacity, fiberglass reinforced plastics (FRP) vessel with manual multi- port valve.
8. Treated water tank: RCC rectangular, (3 x 2 x 2) m, having one centrifugal regenerating pump of 0.75 kW.

11.3 METHODOLOGY AND DATA COLLECTION

Energy consumed during the treatment process is observed to be in the form of electrical, manual, chemical, and mechanical energy. Chemical energy can be considered as indirect energy, human or manual energy as renewable energy and others as non-renewable energy. Each form of energy consumption is calculated in terms of kWh/m^3 of wastewater treated. Primary data have been collected through field monitoring and corroborated with historical data through discussions with plant operators. Log-book and records of transactions and consumptions are also referred for validation. Field monitoring has been done for 15 days spread over 2 months during June–July, 2011. Equal representation of weekdays and weekends is considered for the monitoring days. Time measurement is done using a stopwatch.

11.3.1 ESTIMATION OF ELECTRICAL ENERGY INPUT

The electrical energy input is estimated by considering the electrical load of the pump/motor (kW), time in hours (h) for which the motor is operated and total amount of wastewater treated (Eq. 1).

$$E_p = \frac{P \times T}{Q}$$

where, E_p is the electrical energy kWh/m , Q the total flow of wastewater in m^3/day, P the rated power of the electrical motor in kilo Watt (kW), and T is the operation hours in a day (h/day).

The motor efficiency is assumed as 80 % (Fadare et al. 2010). Table 2 shows the average of values as obtained in the field.

11.3.2 ESTIMATION OF MANUAL ENERGY INPUT

Manual energy is required for different activities on field like operating the switches, opening/closing of the sludge valves, cleaning of the tanks, operating valves to remove the sludge from the tank and collection of sludge in gunny bags to send it to the nearby horticultural garden. Manual energy consumption is a function of the gender of the labor and the nature of activity (Table 3). Based on these considerations, the manual energy is calculated using Eq. 2. The data of field observation (total no. of hours taken to perform the activity) of manual energy are given in Table 4. In the study plant, no female labor is engaged.

$$E_m = \frac{\sum_{i=0}^{i=n}\sum_{j=0}^{j=m} E_{ij} N_{ij} T_{ij}}{Q}$$

where, E_m is manual energy in kWh/m^3, n the number of nature of activities (light, active, and heavy), m the number of gender (male, female), E the human power equivalent (kW), N the number of persons engaged in an activity and T is the total time devoted in the activity (h/day).

11.3.3 ESTIMATION OF FUEL ENERGY

Mechanical energy (E_f) in kWh/m^3 is calculated using Eq. (3)

$$E_f = \frac{15.64D}{Q}$$

where, 15.64 is the unit energy value of diesel in kWh/l (Devi et al. 2007a) and D is the amount of diesel consumed in l/day.

Table 2 Details of mechanical equipment specification

Treatment unit	Type of equipment	No. of working units	P(kW)	T(h/day)
Raw water collection sump	Pump	1	0.75	6.5
Primary treatment	Stirrer	1	0.19	11.75
Chemical dosing tanks	Pump	2	0.19	2.4
RBC treatment	Motor	1	0.19	11.75
Secondary treatment	Stirrer	1	0.19	12.25
	Recirculation pump	1	0.38	5.45
Disinfectant tanks	Pump	2	0.19	2.1
Treated water sump	Pump	1	0.75	5.95

Table 3 Human power equivalent (E) in kW (WHO 1985)

Input	Male	Female	Activities in the treatment plant
Light	0.13	0.10	Switch on/off the raw water pump, maintain the log-book, check motor temperature
Moderate	0.14	0.11	Open/close the sludge drain valve, operation of valves for backwashing,
Heavy	0.54	0.44	Prepare the chemical solution for dosing, fill the chemical solution in the dosing tank, collect the dried sludge in gunny bags

Diesel consumption is found to be 5 l/month for oiling and repairing of machineries.

11.3.4 ESTIMATION OF CHEMICAL ENERGY

Energy is, energy released or absorbed during a chemical reaction. Chemical energy is calculated by estimating the standard enthalpy (heat) of reaction (ΔH) of the chemicals during a reaction.

Chemical energy (E_c) in kWh/m^3 is calculated using Eq. (4)

$$E_c = \frac{n[\Sigma\Delta H_p - \Sigma\Delta H_r]}{Q} \times 0.000278$$

where, n is the number of moles (mol/day), 0.000278 is the conversion factor from KJ to kWh, ΔH_p the enthalpy (heat) of formation of products (kJ/mol), and ΔH_r is enthalpy (heat) of formation of reactants (kJ/mol).

Table 5 shows the chemicals used and their respective quantities for treatment.

11.4 RESULTS AND DISCUSSION

Table 6 gives the assessment of energy consumption pattern in each treatment operation. In addition, the fuel energy (diesel) for entire treatment process is estimated at 0.036 kWh/m^3. Therefore, the total energy consumption is 1.07 kWh/m^3 of wastewater treated. It is much less as compared to the value obtained in a WWTP in California, which was reported to be 1.69 kWh/m^3 excluding manual energy (Stokes and Horvath 2010). There are certain findings that are significant from the point of view of energy planning. First, the electrical form of energy has the biggest share (52 %) of all the forms of energy consumed in the treatment process. However, this is only about half of the total energy consumption. Therefore, electrical energy is not the only form of energy that should be considered in the energy benchmarking exercise. Several studies (for e.g. Devi et al. 2007b; Jonasson 2007; Middlebrooks et al. 1981) have considered only

Table 4 Manual labour input in WWTP

Treatment unit	Nature of activity	Average labour time input (h/day)
Raw water collection sump	Light	0.5
	Medium	-
	Heavy	-
Primary treatment	Light	-
	Medium	1.5
	Heavy	0.5
Chemical dosing tank	Light	2.0
	Medium	-
	Heavy	1.08
RBC treatment	Light	-
	Medium	0.06
	Heavy	0.06
Secondary treatment	Light	-
	Medium	0.28
	Heavy	0.28
Storage tank	Light	-
	Medium	-
	Heavy	0.3
Sludge storage tank	Light	-
	Medium	-
	Heavy	1.25
Sand filter	Light	2
	Medium	-
	Heavy	-
Carbon filter	Light	2
	Medium	-
	Heavy	-

Table 5 Chemicals used in WWTP

Unit	Chemical Name	Form	Quantity
Mixing tank (flocculation)	Caustic soda	Powder	10 g/m^3
	Aluminium sulphate	Powder	10 g/m^3
Treated water tank	Sodium hypo chloride	Liquid	12 ml/m^3

Table 6 Total Energy consumption for the WWTP

Unit	Electrical energy (kWh/m^3)	Manual energy (kWh/m^3)	Chemical energy (kWh/m^3)	Total energy (kWh/m^3)
Sump	0.20	0.003	0.00	0.203
PST	0.09	0.019	0.096	0.205
Dosing tank	0.04	0.046	0.00	0.086
RBC	0.09	0.002	0.00	0.092
SST	0.17	0.008	0.00	0.178
Disinfectant tank	0.03	0.006	0.00	0.036
Sand filter	0.00	0.010	0.00	0.010
Carbon filter	0.00	0.010	0.00	0.010
Treated water tank	0.18	0.00	0.003	0.183
Sludge storage tank	0.00	0.027	0.00	0.027
Total	0.80	0.131	0.099	1.030

the electrical energy and therefore their results do not present the complete energy scenario of a treatment process. The electrical energy consumption per cubic meter of wastewater treatment is found to be 0.80 kWh/m^3. It is commensurate with the findings of several other studies on WWTPs. The values vary in the range of 0.26–0.84 kWh/m^3 (Venkatesh and Brattebo 2011; Pan et al. 2011; Friedrich et al. 2008). The evidences from the literature suggest that the electrical energy consumption can vary by a factor of 1.6 depending upon the choice of the technology and the scale of operation. The major source of electrical energy consumption is in the pump house (79 %) where raw wastewater pumps and treated water pumps have a significant share. Biological treatment process consisting of RBC process consumes 11 % of the total electrical energy consumption.

Second, manual form of energy has the second highest share (32%) during the treatment process. Most of it is used for light work (45%) followed by heavy work (39%). Highest amount of manual energy (35%) is con- sumed during the preparation of chemicals for dosing tank. 21% of manual energy is used for removing the sludge from the sludge tank and disposing to the nearby garden. Looking to the energy pattern of manual energy, it is evident that this form of energy contributes to the total energy consumption and it is inevitable. Third, chemical energy and mechanical energy have insignificant share of 7 and 9%, respectively.

Amongst the treatment processes, the raw water collection sump and primary settling tank consume maximum amount of energy (20%). The energy used here is for pumping the raw water from the sump to the primary settling tank. The disinfectant tank, sand filter and carbon filter account for the least energy consumption. Primary settling tank, secondary settling tank and the treated water tank consume almost the same amount of energy. The treated water tank consumes (18%) as the sump is made below the ground level and secondary settling tank consumes (17%) electrical energy. Dosing tanks and the sludge storage tank consume the highest amount of manual energy of 31 and 21%, respectively. The energy consumed here is for mixing and preparing the chemicals in dosing tanks and removing the dried sludge in gunny bags to the nearest horticulture garden. Primary settling tank uses the highest amount of chemical energy (79%) for flocculation and coagulation. Direct energy has 91% share and renewable energy has 12%.

11.5 CONCLUSIONS

The energy pattern analysis of a small-scale WWTP has been analysed. The energy consumption is found to be about 1.046 kWh/m^3 of wastewater treatment. This is significantly less than the values reported in the literature for large-scale WWTP. Further, previous studies have not included manual energy consumption in their analysis. It is found to be about 32% of the total energy consumption. There is a lot of variation in the reported values in the literature. The plausible reason is that the energy intensity depends on the capacity of the treatment plant, extent of automation, and choice of treatment technology. This suggests that a number of such investigations are required for various categories of treatment plants so as to have a holistic view on the wastewater treatment and energy-nexus. Based on the evidence of this study, it can be stated that the decentralized treatment systems have less energy intensity in comparison to a large-scale plant. This could be partly attributable to the use of manual energy in the treatment process in a small-scale plant. However, such a generalization needs to be supported with a number of analyses for various types of treatment processes and wastewater characterization in various regions of the world.

REFERENCES

1. Devi R, Dahiya RP, Kumar A, Singh V (2007a) Meeting energy requirement of wastewater treatment in rural sector. Energy policy 35:3891–3897
2. Devi R, Singh V, Dahiya RP, Kumar A (2007b) Energy consumption pattern of a decentralized community in northern Haryana. Renew Sustain Energy Rev 13:194–200
3. Fadare DA, Nkpubre DO, Oni AO, Falana A, Waheed MA, Bamiro OA (2010) Energy and exergy analyses of malt drink production in Nigeria. Energy 35:5336–5346
4. Food and Agriculture Organization, World Health Organization, and United Nations University (FAO/WHO/UNU) (1985) Energy and Protein Requirements. Report of Joint FAO/WHO/UNU Expert Consultation. WHO Technical Report Series No. 724. Geneva: World Health Organization
5. Friedrich E, Pillay S, Buckley CA (2008). Environmental life-cycle assessments for water treatment processes—a South African case study of an urban water cycle. http://www.assaf.co.za/wp- content/uploads/2010/04/WaterSAJan09.pdf Appl Water Sci (2012) 2:221–226
6. Hellstrom D (1997) An exergy analysis for a wastewater treatment plant: an estimation of the consumption of physical resources. Water Environ Res 69(1):44–51

7. Jonasson M (2007) Energy benchmark for wastewater treatment process—a comparison between Sweden and Austria. Dissertation. Department of Industrial Electrical Engineering and Automation, Lund University, Lund
8. Mahgoub M, El SM, Steen NPVD, Zeid KA, Vairavamoorthy K (2010) Towards sustainability in urban water: a life cycle analysis of the urban water system of Alexandria City, Egypt. J Clean Prod 18:1100–1006
9. Merlin G, Lissolo T (2010) Energy and exergy analysis to evaluate sustainability of small wastewater treatment plants: application to a constructed wetland and a sequencing batch reactor. J Water Resour Prot 2:997–1009
10. Middlebrooks E, Middlebrooks H, Reed S (1981) Energy requirement for small wastewater treatment systems. Water Pollut control Fed 53(7):1172–1197
11. Pan T, Zhu D-X, Ye P-Y (2011) Estimate of life-cycle greenhouse gas emissions from a vertical subsurface flow constructed wetland and conventional wastewater treatment plants: a case study in China. Ecol Eng 37:248–254
12. Stokes RJ, Horvath A (2010) Supply chain environmental effects of wastewater utilities. Environ Res Lett 5:014015 (7 pp)
13. Venkatesh G, Brattebo H (2011) Energy consumption, costs and environmental impacts for urban water cycle services: case study of Oslo (Norway). Energy 36:792–800

PART VI

CONCLUSION

CHAPTER 12

Sustainable Urban (re-)Development with Building Integrated Energy, Water and Waste Systems

THORSTEN SCHUETZE, JOONG-WON LEE, AND TAE-GOO LEE

12.1 INTRODUCTION

Growing urbanization, increasing resource consumption, and limited resource availability mean that urban user behavior and infrastructure systems need to be transformed to become more efficient and for a more sustainable use and management of resources, particularly for the provision of primary services such as energy, water and food.

Our present civilization is to a large extent based on principles of centralization. The large technical effort for the construction, service, and maintenance of centralized infrastructure systems and the related processes involves high monetary and environmental costs endured by society. The dissipation caused by conventional centralized infrastructure systems is similar for energy, water supply and wastewater discharge. For example, almost 70% of the primary energy required for centralized electricity production in conventional power plants is lost. The building sector is responsible worldwide for more than 33% of the total resources and 40% of the total energy consumption [1]. The burning of fossil energy carriers contributes to most of the anthropogenic CO_2 emissions. The conventional global food production is responsible for most of the anthropogenic freshwater consumption, a large component of the global CO_2 emissions (from soil carbon losses and chemical fertilizer production) and energy consumption for farming, harvesting, storage, and transport of agricultural products.

Particularly relevant is the negative interrelationship between urban and rural areas. The decoupling of food and drinking water production and wastewater management results in the pollution of natural sources of livelihood and the elimination of resources. In contrast, sustainable infrastructure systems, based on the principles of circular flow economy, involve the efficient and local use and reuse of resources.

Many of the world‘s cities are expected to grow significantly during the following decades. While currently already more than 50% of the world‘s population lives in cities, it is expected that this percentage will grow to approximately 60%, with a yearly rate of 1.7% until 2030. Accordingly, the world faces a rural exodus and shrinking rural population as the urbanization rate exceeds the global population growth. In the framework of this urbanization process, 37 urban agglomerations are expected to become mega cities by 2025 [2].

Similar to rural area residents, many people dwelling in smaller cities will need to deal with the phenomenon of population shrinkage, particularly in countries with low birth and immigration rates, such as most European countries as well as Korea and Japan. Both of these situations put pressure on the operation and management of conventional centralized infrastructure systems for energy and water and organic waste management. The disadvantages of these systems include the lockup of capital for very long periods, limitations in provision and discharge such as the mixing of sewage streams with different noxious factors (being a barrier for appropriate treatment and reuse), the supply of drinking water only, and the in-adaptability to changing demographic structures and quantities, as well as high monetary costs. In contrast with such large-scale centralized infrastructures, the building integration of decentralized infrastructures for energy, water, and organic waste management has many advantages

[3–6]. Furthermore, appropriate system approaches for supply, efficient use, treatment, recycling, and reuse facilitate the realization of so called zero-emission buildings.

However, the term "zero-emission" is generally associated with the reduction of specific emissions, particularly greenhouse gases such as CO_2 caused by the burning of fossil energy carriers for the generation and provision of thermal and electrical energy, such as by the use of renewable energy. For example, in 2009 in Milan, Italy, the Milano Scala, a self-declared zero-emission hotel, was established [7]. The concept includes the use of efficient electric devices for the provision of heating and cooling energy and the required electric energy originates from clean sources and therefore does not cause pollution at local and global levels. Additionally, water efficient technologies are applied. The building has achieved 2 of the 3 maximum available "tents", an award of the "ecoluxury" certification, which is provided by a collaboration of ecologically and socially responsible businesses in the luxury tourism sector [8]. Buildings aiming for zero-emission should not produce any harmful emissions but on the contrary, produce energy, water, and resources. Such an integrated approach was taken in the development for a youth center with seminar facilities and a restaurant in Berlin, Germany. The concept is based on the building integration of new and innovative technologies and systems, which have been proven in practice in different pilot projects. In the framework of this paper, the overall systems approach will be discussed, as well as the different sub-systems and technologies.

12.2 OBJECTIVES AND METHODOLOGY

This article discusses the latest results from the authors' own investigation into the decentralized and building integrated management of energy, water, and organic waste in relation to the sustainable development of new and existing cities. The case studies presented act as examples of the applied research in integrated urban resource management in Germany, from the latest theories to selected detailed examples. This paper describes the most recent developments in decentralized technologies in, and system approaches towards, self-sufficient buildings with zero emissions. It aims to identify, examine, and demonstrate the effectiveness of decentralized systems approaches for energy, water, and organic waste management that face the latest challenges identified for the future design of urban infrastructures. Mainly based on the effective use, reuse, and production of energy, water, and organic waste as well as on the separation of sewage streams with different properties, the insights from case studies serve to prove the applicability of those approaches. Quantitative data on water and nutrient flows from specific case studies were collected, while qualitative analysis of approved resource management concepts was carried out based on recent research findings and the authors' own inquiries. Finally, the application of building integrated systems for the management of water, organic waste, and energy emerges as the appropriate procedure for the sustainable transition of conventional urban infrastructures for the management of these resources. The integrated concept for building integrated resource management in a youth center in Berlin, Germany was examined in terms of the applicability and a way forward for sustainable urban (re-)development.

The building integration of appropriate infrastructure systems for energy, water, and organic waste management can facilitate the realization of zero-emission buildings and can contribute to the sustainable development of new—or the redevelopment of existing—urban areas and cities. This approach has been successfully implemented in the concept of a new youth center (Figure 1) with accommodation and seminar facilities in Berlin, Germany (subsequently referred as "Berlin youth center"). The building owner is the registered —Ludwig-Wolker-Haus‖ association. The specific objectives of the project are:

- Reduction of the direct water footprint to the greatest possible degree through on-site Water Supply and Waste Water Management according to the principles of Integrated Water Resource Management. Minimization of fresh water demand by approximately 50% through the application of water efficient systems, the collection, processing and recycling of wastewater, rainwater harvesting and utilization for non-drinking purposes, and the augmentation of freshwater bodies.

- Operation of an organic waste free building through the collection of human urine and reuse as fertilizer, the collection of solids from black water and organic waste for fermentation and composting processing, and the subsequent local use of black fertile soil produced in horticulture and agriculture (for the production of food and renewable energy).
- Net zero energy consumption through minimization of the building‘s service energy demand, local production, and the efficient utilization, storage and export of surplus energy into external grids which also serve as energy providers in periods of need.
- No additional building and service costs in comparison with reference buildings through smart and integrated design and planning as well as savings in centralized infrastructure systems and conventional service costs.

12.3 RESULTS AND DISCUSSION

Integrated urban water resource management, including rainwater harvesting, the recycling of wastewater, as well as the recovery of nutrients and the processing of organic waste is essential for sustainable urban development and shows considerable potential for (urban) agriculture, but is as yet relatively underutilized. "Meanwhile, good agriculture and forestry practices can contribute to sound watershed management, safeguarding water catchment and reducing runoff and flooding in cities-ever more important as climate change increases the frequency of extreme weather events" [9].

12.3.1 REDUCTION OF THE DIRECT WATER FOOTPRINT

Extensive quantities of water could be saved with technologies that allow for fresh water savings and water recycling. The first step for the reduction of water consumption is the installation of water saving toilets, showerheads, and taps, which for example allow a reduction of household freshwater consumption of approximately 30% without loss of comfort [4,5]. Such water saving measures are achievable without additional costs if they are installed in the framework of new installations in place of standard appliances. The Berlin youth center will be equipped with water saving taps (with flow rates of 3 liters per min), showerheads (with flow rates of less than 5 liters per min) and toilets (with flush volumes of 2 and 3.5 liters per flush). Additional savings will be achieved with the collection of rainwater and so-called "greywater" from showers and bathtubs and its decentralized recycling in the basement of the building. By means of water saving measures, the recycling of greywater and reuse in form of so-called service water for non-drinking purpose, the water consumption and related fees can be reduced by approximately 50% compared with standard water installations. Due to savings in drinking water fees (2,169 Euros per m^3 including VAT) and sewage fees (2,464 Euros per m^3 including VAT) which can be achieved in Berlin by reduced drinking water consumption [10], it is expected that the water system for the reduction of the direct water footprint in the Berlin youth center will be economically profitable. In comparison with the business as usual option, the operating savings of the described water system are expected to be sufficient to cover the service costs and initial capital costs.

The service water will be used for toilet flush and irrigation of the green roof and garden. Surplus water will be infiltrated and recharge the groundwater. The advantage of the decentralized collection and processing of greywater and the direct reuse at the building level is the comparable small infrastructure, consisting of collection and supply pipes, which is required for its installation. Compared with the overall system costs and the achievable savings, the costs for such a system are comparatively low [4]. Furthermore, the system offers the potential for recycling of energy as will be further discussed subsequently.

By as early as 1996, Europe‘s first economically profitable large-scale greywater recycling facility was realized in a four star hotel in Offenbach/Main (Germany). The installation of the greywater recycling facility for 400 guests only occupies the equivalent space of two car-parking places in the underground parking lot of the hotel. The recycled water is used in the hotel for flushing the toilets and the surplus is used for irrigation. The payback period for the 72,000 Euros investment, operation, service

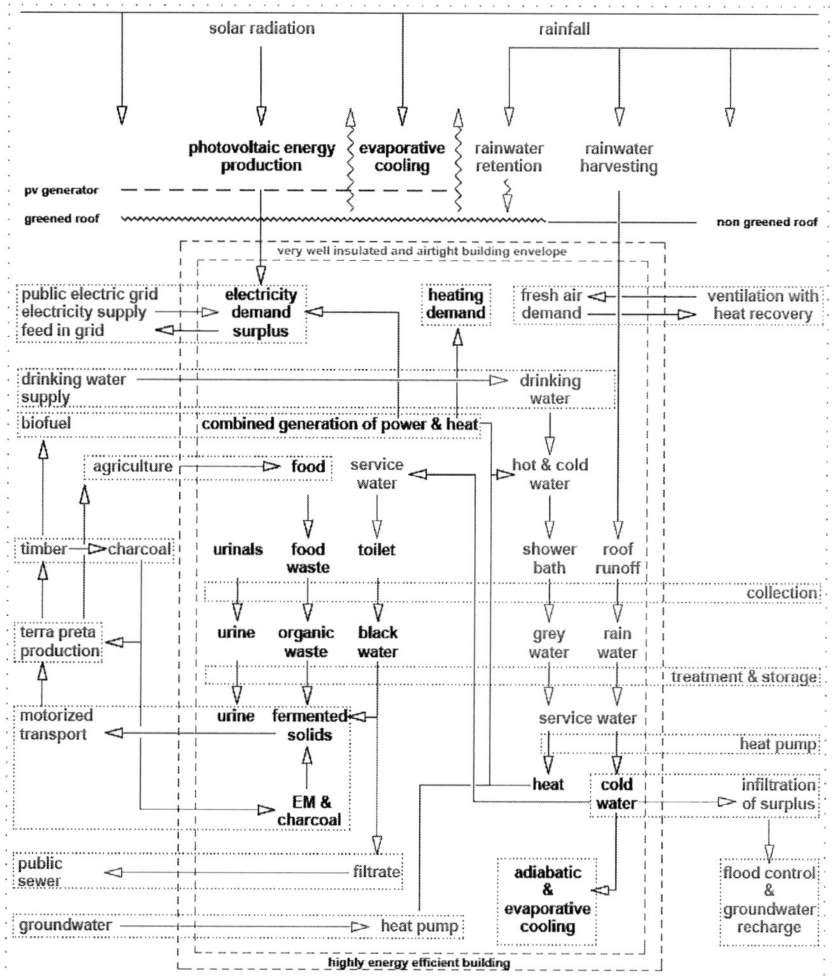

Figure 1. Simplified diagram of the overall systems approach discussed in the framework of this paper. External and building integrated sub-systems and technologies for the sustainable management of energy, water and organic waste are briefly described by showing their relationship to each other as well as the connecting flows.

and maintenance costs was only 6.5 years. Accordingly, the system has been economically profitable for more than 8 years. On average, 3,700 m^3 of drinking water could be saved per year, resulting in savings of 18,500 Euros in drinking water and sewage fees (which are in Offenbach approximately 5 Euros/m^3). The electric energy consumption of the greywater recycling facility including the distribution of service water is approx. 1.5 kWh. Over the past 15 years, since the installation of the described facility, the technology of greywater recycling facilities has been further developed, resulting in lower system costs and enhanced control and monitoring systems. The monitoring and control of contemporary facilities for water recycling can be executed by the company that also builds and installs the facility, therefore providing an overall integrated service [11].

In the case of the Berlin youth center, all greywater and rainwater will be managed on the property. It is expected that the investment service and maintenance costs for the decentralized rainwater management system will be covered by savings in drinking water and sewage fees, and the yearly fee of 1.897 Euros per m^2 property draining in the sewerage system of Berlin [10]. The small amount of sludge originating from the biological greywater treatment process will be collected and processed together with the separated solids from blackwater (sewage originating from toilets) processing and collected organic wastes.

12.3.2 MANAGEMENT OF ORGANIC WASTE AND NUTRIENTS USING THE EXAMPLE OF CASE STUDIES

In the Berlin youth center, blackwater will be collected separately and filtrated in the basement of the building to recover the majority of the contained organic solids and nutrients. These substances can be used as resources for the production of fertile black soil to be reused in urban horticulture and agriculture. The remaining filtrate has a reduced pollution load and is easier to clean than untreated effluent from toilets. For example, in a public toilet facility in a central train station of the city of Hamburg (subsequently referred as "Hamburg toilet facility"), separated blackwater drainage, filtration, and a solid collection system have been successfully installed and operated since 2010. In the same facility, waterless urinals are also installed, facilitating the separate collection of undiluted urine for the purposes of both the reuse as liquid fertilizer and the reduction of the pollutant load of sewage streams. The experiences and findings from the separated urine and blackwater collection and treatment systems in the Hamburg toilet facility are also used for the planning and system optimization of the blackwater and organic waste processing system which will be installed in the Berlin youth center.

The separated solids (mainly feces and toilet paper) are transported automatically to a storage tank where they are mixed with a specific portion of vegetal charcoal powder (also known as "bio char") and liquid Effective Microorganisms (EM). The mixture of these ingredients causes a lactic acid fermentation process that has already started during the intermediate anaerobic storage in the container. No gas or malodor is emitted. Full containers are transported to a facility for the production of anthropogenic fertile black soil also known as "Terra Preta" (Portuguese: Black Soil). In 2011, parts of the collected and fermented solids were transported to the Botanical Gardens in Berlin (Germany) where they were used in the framework of the Terraboga research project [12] for the production of Terra Preta and its use in urban agriculture.

The Terraboga research project is built on the findings that the production of anthropogenic black soil (which has been originally produced by cultures in the Brazilian Amazon basin) is based on a lactic acid fermentation process which incorporates manure from humans and/or animals, organic material, as well as vegetable charcoal. The nutrients (mainly Nitrogen and Phosphorous) contained in the feces are bound to the charcoal particles and are locked until they are made available to the roots of plants by microorganisms. Therefore, Terra Preta facilitates the cultivation of plants in nutrient rich soil whereby the addition of artificial fertilizers is not required. Even though such soil is rich in nutrients, it could contribute to the purification of rainwater runoff, also in the case of heavy precipitation events. The good water storage facilities could help to cope with floods and periods of drought and could therefore be used for the adaptation to the effects of climate change. Furthermore, by utilizing vegetable charcoal in the soil, carbon can be stored (in contrast to soils which are used for conventional agriculture that release carbon to the atmosphere).

Therefore, the application of Terra Preta could contribute to the mitigation of climate change [13].

In both cases of the Hamburg toilet facility and the Berlin youth center, the remaining filtrate from the blackwater separation process is discharged to the public sewer systems. While the filtrate should preferably also be treated on-site and be reused, due to the comparable small quantity, the related effort and mandatory requirement to connect the drainage systems to the public sewer system, it has been decided to discharge the filtered blackwater to the sewer system [14].

Depending on the amount of separated urine, it is estimated that more than 50% of the total Phosphorous and 10% of the total Nitrogen contained in the wastewater stream of the Berlin youth center can be collected and processed for reuse in fertile black soil. In the Berlin youth center, the filtered solids from blackwater will be collected in containers and pre-fermented with charcoal and EM together with the organic wastes from the restaurant. Effective recycling management and the link between organic waste and energy production is realized by applying Terra Preta for the cultivation of fast growing timber. This timber can be used for combined heat and power generation and the production of charcoal, which can then be reused in the previously described concept. It is planned to use Terra Preta for the enhancement of soils in urban horticulture not meant for human consumption (such as in parks and gardens), because there are concerns regarding the security of food grown with Terra Preta made from human feces. Terra Preta use for the cultivation of fast growing timber would facilitate the production of renewable energy carriers in the form of biomass.

To reduce the drinking water consumption and to facilitate the reuse of precious nutrients in human urine (yellow water), waterless urinals for the separate collection of urine will be installed in the men‘s toilets assigned to the restaurant and conference facilities. The undiluted urine will be collected by means of a separate drainage pipe system and stored intermediately in containers located in the basement of the hotel building. At specific intervals, the filled urine containers will be replaced by empty containers and transported to a central treatment facility for further processing and reuse as fertilizer or to produce nutrient enriched fertile black soil. Experiences with undiluted urine collection show that in drainage systems with open ventilation pipes, approximately 50% of the ammonia contained in urine evaporates and gets lost through the ventilation system [15]. The yellow water collection and storage system for the Berlin youth center will therefore be equipped with a newly developed and enhanced drainage and collection system which facilitates the reduction of ammonia evaporation losses.

The separated collection of urine offers considerable potential for pollution control, resource recovery, and the optimization of existing wastewater management systems because it contains up to 90% of the total Nitrogen and 50% of the Phosphorous as well as a large portion of the micro pollutants in domestic sewage. The separation of those nutrients enhances the efficiency of conventional sewage treatment processes and facilitates their reuse as fertilizer in agriculture [16]. The eco toxicological effect of human medicines in domestic wastewater (so called micro pollutants) could be reduced by 50% [17], and the part separation of urine could turn wastewater treatment plants from energy consumers to energy producers [18]. The experiences with building integrated urine separation systems show that waterless urinals work well, emit no malodor, and are convenient to use; however, functionality of the separation with so-called "separation" or "no-mix" toilets is still insufficient [19]. For an optimal operation, a close collaboration with the maintenance service provider proved to be a critical factor for optimal operation in the framework of a three-year operation and monitoring phase of no-mix toilets in the "Forum Chriesbach" in Switzerland [15]. Furthermore, the water consumption of available separation toilets (with 6 liters per flush) is similar to conventional water saving toilets. Therefore, in the investigated Hamburg toilet facility and the Berlin youth center rather than separation toilets, water saving toilets with maximum flush volumes of only 3.5 liters will be installed.

While the greywater recycling system in the Berlin youth center is expected to be economically profitable, because the operating savings will exceed the initial capital and service costs in less than 7 years, the separated collection and processing of or urine and blackwater with organic waste will produce additional service costs, because there is no market yet for products such as fertilizer and soil made from urine and blackwater. In comparison with the business-as-usual option, the operating savings of such a resource productive sanitation system are expected to be not sufficient to cover the service costs and initial capital costs. Therefore, this matter is being investigated in the framework of on-going research projects, such as for example in Terraboga, which examines how such productive sanitation systems can be integrated in suitable fee systems for circular flow economies. However, according to experiences in the Hamburg toilet facility and cost benefit calculations executed in the framework of the Terraboga project, the monetary savings in drinking water and sewage fees (compared with standard water and sanitary installations) can cover the additional construction costs of such decentralized collection and treatment systems.

12.3.3 ENERGY EFFICIENCY AND PRODUCTIVITY

The Berlin youth center is planned as "lowest-energy-building" with minimized energy demand for heating, cooling, and warm water production. The electricity demand for the operation of the building will be significantly reduced to limit the primary energy consumption for the operation of the hotel to 120 kW/m^{2}a. Low heating energy and Passive House concepts are transferable to commercial buildings and a primary energy consumption of less than 100 kWh/m^{2}a can be achieved without extra investment costs compared to conventional office buildings [20].

To realize a building with net zero energy consumption, the remaining primary energy demand must be produced on the building by means of renewable energy sources. The most common means for this purpose are building integrated photovoltaic generators as well as combined heat and power generators that use renewable fuels. By 2010, more than 300 building projects worldwide have been realized (mainly in Europe) which aimed to achieve a net-zero energy balance [21].

According to the European Energy in Buildings Performance Directive, by 2021 all new buildings in the EU must be built as nearly zero energy buildings with an energy demand of "zero" or "nearly zero" for heating, cooling, and hot water production; for public buildings, this must be achieved by 2019. The remaining energy demand must be produced to a very significant degree on the building or in the direct neighborhood by means of renewable energy sources. Also, in the framework of renovation of the existing building stock, important measures for enhancing the energy efficiency are required [22]. Accordingly, from 2020 all new building projects should be almost energy neutral and regarding the consumption of non-renewable energy resources already nearly zero-energy buildings.

The measures, which will be taken to achieve good energy efficiency, are a well-insulated building envelope, the reduction of thermal bridges, and the installation of a mechanical ventilation system with heat recovery. As these measures are quite common for energy efficient buildings, new and innovative measures for energy efficiency will also be applied that are based on the creation of synergies between the water and energy sectors.

For example, the previously described facility for the recycling of greywater will be used in the Berlin youth center for the recovery of heat. A pilot installation of the so-called "Pontos Heat Cycle" in student apartments still operates properly and has been monitored for a period of two years. The evaluation results indicate that monetary and energy savings are more profitable when greywater is combined with heat recovery. By using two heat exchangers, the cold freshwater is pre-heated by the comparable warm greywater. On a yearly average, approximately 20% less energy is required for hot water production compared with systems without heat recovery [23]. To enhance the energy efficiency of the heat recovery system, the greywater recycling facility for the Berlin youth center has a different system layout. The greywater will be collected and purified in a thermally insulated recycling facility. The resulting hot service water will be used as a heat source for a heat pump, which will facilitate a much higher heat recovery rate than the Pontos Heat Cycle. In comparison with a business-as-usual solution, the operating savings of such an integrated water recycling and heat recovery facility are expected to exceed the service cost and initial capital costs.

It is expected that the greatest portion of the hot water demand can be supplied by heat extraction from purified grey water. The cooled service water is stored in a thermally insulated tank that serves as a heat sink for the building's adiabatic cooling system. During the hot summer periods, when cooling may be required to provide comfortable indoor temperatures, the cold water can be used for the building component activation of floor slabs. Also, the use of purified grey water for irrigation and evaporation on the building‘s greened roof will contribute to cooling. Additional service water will be provided by means of rainwater harvesting from non-greened roof surfaces and utilization, collected from the non-greened roof surfaces. The evaporation cooling on the roof also creates synergies with photovoltaic energy production.

Photovoltaic generators will be installed on the flat roof of the building. Synergies between the photovoltaic energy production and the evaporative cooling with service water can be achieved on the greened roof areas. Due to the significant lower temperature of the intensively irrigated greened roof, the PV modules are expected to have a higher efficiency of 8–10% during hot summer days in comparison with modules, which are installed on conventional roofs (without evaporative cooling). Due to the comparable small roof surface area of the hotel, the PV modules can only contribute partly to the renewable production of the energy required for the building service. As the Berlin youth center is located in the city center and surrounded by relatively high buildings, the installation of Photovoltaic modules on the façades of the building was not regarded as productive.

Another renewable energy source that can be used is near-surface geothermal energy, which is extracted from the ground under the building. Since near-surface geothermal energy (up to a depth of 100 m) is actually stored solar energy, it is indeed renewable. Most of the hotel's remaining thermal and electrical energy demand during the winter will be covered by a biogas driven combined heat and power (CHP) generator. In the future the gas burner is planned to be replaced with a CHP that can burn solid biofuels such as fast grown timber originating from regional plantations and fertile black soil originating from the building‘s own organic wastes. A regional recycling economy could thus be realized. Technologies that facilitate the production of thermal and electric energy as well as vegetable charcoal at the same time, are not yet available but are in the focus of research projects executed by producers of CHP generators [24]. Such technology would indeed facilitate the creation of synergies between sustainable organic waste management, sanitation, food, and energy production, and would therefore prepare the ground for sustainable development.

12.4 CONCLUSIONS AND OUTLOOK

The application of building integrated sustainable infrastructure systems, which have been discussed in the framework of this paper can contribute significantly to both sustainable urban and rural development. According to the presented research findings, the direct water footprint of buildings can be reduced by 50% through water use efficiency and recycling measures. Furthermore, rainwater can be managed on building and property level by means of retention, harvesting, collection, utilization, evaporation and infiltration. The construction, service and maintenance of efficient water use, reuse and rainwater management systems can be realized with available technologies and, in the German cases, without additional costs compared with conventional water and sanitation systems, due to achievable monetary savings in drinking water-, sewage- and stormwater-fee. In comparison with a business as usual solution, the operating savings of such sustainable water management systems can cover the initial capital costs.

According to the experiences of the Hamburg toilet facility, the cost for the installation of decentralized urine collection and blackwater treatment systems can be covered in part by savings in drinkwater and sewage fee, which can be achieved by the installation of water saving toilets and waterless urinals. Regarding the cost and benefits for the operation, transport, and processing of human excreta together with organic waste for the production of Terra Preta, no evaluation of the economic data is yet available. However, it can be expected that the described system is not economically profitable in the current state, since the technology is still in development and there is no market yet for Terra Preta. In comparison with a business as usual solution, the operating savings of the described productive sanitation systems in the specific German cases could not cover the initial capital costs.

Nearly Zero Energy Buildings Energy can be realized by construction of energy efficient buildings and the renewable production of the remaining energy demand on building level, for example with solar thermal collectors and Photovoltaic (PV) generators. Worldwide a considerable amount of such buildings has been realized. It can be expected that zero energy buildings will be built with growing tendency and will become a common building type in many countries. In the EU regulation new buildings have to be built as nearly zero energy buildings by 2020 [22]. According to the Presidential Committee on Green Growth also in the Republic of Korea new buildings have to be build from 2025 as zero energy houses with an energy saving rate of 100% [25]. Declining costs for decentralized produced electricity with PV support the trend towards zero energy buildings. Countries with higher electricity consumer prices, such as Germany and Denmark reached already "socket parity" in 2012 while countries with lower electricity consumer prices are expected to reach socket parity in the coming years, e.g., France and Turkey in 2015 and the Republic of Korea in 2017. 'Socket parity' is defined in this case "as the point where a household can make 5% or more return on investment in a PV system just by using the energy generated to replace household energy consumption" [26]. Accordingly the decentralized production of electricity with Photovoltaic is in the German case economically profitable because the operating savings can cover and exceed the initial capital costs.

The transferability of the results presented in this paper, particularly regarding economical aspects and the decentralized management of rainwater are limited to environments, whose basic conditions are similar to the German case studies. The effort and the related costs for the decentralized management of rainwater can vary significantly depending on the local climate and soil properties. The balance of monetary costs and achievable savings for decentralized water and energy systems is for example heavily dependent on the specific fee levels and structures for the discharge of rainwater and domestic sewage, and the consumption of drinking water and energy.

High fee levels and specific fee structures encourage decentralized management of rainwater and sustainable water use. In Berlin for example 4.63 Euros/m^3 can be saved in sewage and drinking water fees per cubic meter drinking water [10]. In contrast, low fee levels inhibit efficient and sustainable water use. In the city of Seoul in the Republic of Korea the sum of the drinking water and sewage per m^3 ranges from 450 Won (approximately 0.31 Euros for public bath), over 480 Won (approx. 0.33 Euros for household) and 730 Won (approx. 0.50 Euros for business) and 970 Won (approx. 0.67 Euros for commercial) [27]. Accordingly, the achievable savings by efficient water use in Berlin are, depending on the building type, between 7 to 15 times higher than in Seoul. Therefore, the investment in sustainable water management is regarding economical aspects in Berlin more attractive than it is in Seoul. However, specific aspects of sustainable water management are stimulated in the Republic of Korea by other means, such as legislations and tax reductions. According to the national water act, which is in effect since 2003, hotels, shopping malls and industries with specific water consumption have for example to install wastewater recycling facilities and reuse the water for non-drinking purpose such irrigation and toilet flush. The government subsidizes the investment costs through tax reductions [28].

Resource dependency, particularly regarding energy, food, and fresh water can be significantly reduced by an area wide application of building integrated sustainable infrastructure systems and the creation of synergies between different sectors, such as water, energy and organic waste. A circular flow economy could be introduced for growing and shrinking cities by decentralization, participation, and resource intelligence. This would result in lower construction, service, and maintenance costs and the protection of the environment and natural resources. Particularly, the large Korean and Asian market for the construction of new towns and cities that aim to be sustainable and "green," shows considerable potential for the application of such decentralized zero-emission concepts.

However, the worldwide development of integrated concepts for the green and sustainable (re-)development of rural and urban areas which are not based on conventional centralized infrastructure systems for energy and water supply, wastewater, organic waste management, and food production is still at its beginning stage. Therefore, further theoretical and applied research and development in the framework of pilot projects, and the dissemination of the results, is crucial to enhance public awareness, international and national recognition, and to introduce a paradigm shift in the design, construction, and operation of urban and rural infrastructure systems.

The first author of this paper is coordinating the research project ZEB-ISTIS Zero Emission Building-Integrating Sustainable Technologies and

Infrastructure Systems supported by the KORANET Korean scientific co-operation network with the European Research Area, joint call on Green Technologies [29]. The aim of the project which will run until autumn 2014 is the further development and optimization of sustainable building integrated infrastructure systems, including the integration and creation of synergies between social, environmental and economical aspects. Furthermore, the project will contribute to the knowledge transfer between the partners form Korea and Europe (Germany, Switzerland, Turkey) and the dissemination of information for the adapted design, planning, operation and maintenance of Zero Emission Buildings.

REFERENCES

1. UNEP. Buildings and Climate Change Summary for Decision-Makers; UNEP DTIE Sustainable Consumption and Production Branch: Paris, France, 2009; p. 62.
2. United Nations, D.o.E.a.S.A. Population Division World Urbanization Prospects, the 2011 Revision; United Nations Department of Economic and Social Affairs/ Population Division: New York, NY, USA, 2012; p. 318.
3. DWA Deutsche Vereinigung fur Wasserwirtschaft, A.u. A.e.V. Neuartige Sanitärsysteme, 1sted.; DWA: Hennef, Germany, 2008; Volume 1, p. 333.
4. Schuetze, T. Dezentrale Wassersysteme im Wohnungsbau internationalerGroßstädte am Beispiel der Städte Hamburg in Deutschland und Seoul in Sud-Korea; Books on Demand: Norderstedt, Germany, 2005; p. 496.
5. Schuetze, T.; Tjallingi, S.P.; Correlje, A.; Ryu, M.; Graaf, R.; van der Ven, F. Every Drop Counts: Environmentally Sound Technologies for Urban and Domestic Water Use Efficiency, 1st ed.; United Nations Environment Programme: Nairobi, Kenya, 2008; p.197.
6. Binz, C.; Larsen, C.; Maurer, M.; Truffer, B.; Gebauer, H. Zukunft der dezentralen Wassertechnologien; EAWAG: Dubendorf, Switzerland, 2010; p. 59.
7. Hotel-Milano-Scala Eco Sustainability—The first zero-emissions hotel in Milan. Available online: http://www.hotelmilanoscala.it/en/milan-hotel-eco-sustainability/ (accessed on 31 December 2012).
8. Ecoluxury. The Ecolouxury Philosophy. Available online: http://www.ecoluxury.com/en/ philosophy.php/ (accessed on 15 May 2012).
9. FAO. Innovations in water management needed to sustain cities. Available online: http://www.fao.org/news/story/en/item/53479/icode/ (accessed on 31 December 2012).
10. Berliner Wasserbetriebe Unsere Tarife. Available online: http://www.bwb.de/content/language1/ html/204.php/ (accessed on 27 January 2012).
11. Kionka, T. Wasser, jeder Liter zählt. Grauwasser-Recycling in Hotels. MGT—Moderne Gebäudetechnik 2008, 62, 10–13.

12. Berlin, F. Terraboga. Available online: http://www.terraboga.de/ (accessed on 1 January 2013).
13. Factura,H.;Bettendorf,T.;Buzie,C.;Pieplow,H.;Reckin,J.;Otterpohl,R.TerraPretasanitation: Re-discovered from an ancient Amazonian civilisation—Integrating Sanitation, Bio-waste management and agriculture. Water Sci. Technol. 2010, 61, 2673–2679.
14. Thomas, P. TerraBoGa-Zwischenbericht der HATI GmbH; HATI GmbH: Berlin, Germany, 2011; p. 39.
15. Goosse, P. NoMix Toilettensystem. GWA Magazin 2009, 7, 567–574.
16. Schuetze, T.; van Loosdrecht, M.M. Urine Separation for Sustainable Urban Water-Management. In Water Infrastructure for Sustainable Communities—China and The World; Hao, X., Novotny, V., Nelson, V., Eds.; IWA Publishing: London, UK, 2010; pp. 213–225. Sustainability 2013, 5 1127
17. Larsen, T.A.; Lienert, J. Final Report Novaquatis. NoMix—A New Approach to Urban Water Management; EAWAG: Dübendorf, Switzerland, 2007; p. 32.
18. Wilsenach, J.; van Loosdrecht, M. Integration of Processes to Treat Wastewater and Source-Separated Urine. J. Environ. Eng. 2006, 132, 11.
19. Luthi, C.; Panesar, A.; Schutze, T.; Norström, A.; McConville, J.; Parkinson, J.; Saywell, D.; Ingle, R. Sustainable Sanitation in Cities—A Framework for Action, 1st ed.; Papiroz Publishing House: The Hague, The Netherlands, 2011; Volume 1, p. 169.
20. Löhnert, G .EnOB Energy Efficiency in Commercial Buildings.Experiences and Results from the German Funding Programme Energy Optimized Building EnOB. In Zero Enery Building Workshop 2012; Fraunhofer Representative Office Korea: Energy Dream Center, Seoul, Korea, 2012.
21. Musall, E.; Weiss, T.; Lenoir, A.; Voss, K.; Garde, F.; Donn, M. Net Zero energy solar buildings: An overview and analysis on worldwide building projects. In EuroSun 2010; International Solar Energy Society (ISES) IEA Solar Heating & Cooling Programme (SHC): Graz, Austria, 2010.
22. European Parliament and the Council of the European Union. Directive 2010/31/EU of the European Parliament and of the Council of 19 May 2010 on the energy performance of buildings. In European Parliament and the Council of the European Union: Brussels, Belgium, 2010; p. 23.
23. Vetter, C. Wärmerückgewinnung aus Grauwasser mit dem Pontos Heat Cycle.In-Wasserautarkes Grundstück; Fachvereinigung Betriebsund Regenwassernutzung e.V.: Darmstadt, Germany, 2011; Volume 15, pp. 63–78.
24. DK, S. Research and development project of pyrolysis based combustion system. Available online: http://stirling.dk/page_content.php?menu_id=30&type=submenu/ (accessed on 1 January 2013).
25. Chun, S. Korean Energy Management Cooperation, Building Energy Policies in Korea. In International Workshop EPC (Energy Performance Certificate) and Assessor System for Buildings; Korean Energy Management Cooperation: Seoul Olympic Parktel, Seoul, Korea, 2012.
26. Baziliana, M.; Onyejia, I.; Liebreichd, M.; MacGille, I.; Chased, J.; Shahf, J.; Gieleng, D.; Arenth, D.; Landfeari, D.; Zhengrongj, S. Re-considering the economics of photovoltaic power. Renew. Energ. 2013, 53, 329–338.

27. Seoul Metropolitean Government Arisu—The office of Waterworks Seoul Metropolitean Government, Information on Water and Sewage Billing in English. Available online:http://water.seoul.go.kr/sudohome/english/bill_gallery.php/ (accessed on 27 February 2013).
28. Ministry of Environment Republic of Korea Green Korea 2001; Ministry of Environment Republic of Korea: Seoul, Korea, 2001; p. 77.
29. Heinrichs, G.; Westphal, H. Korean scientific cooperation network with the European Research Area—2012 Joint Call on Green Technologies. Available online: http://www.koranet.eu/en/229.php/ (accessed on 1 February 2013).

CHAPTER 13

Urban Ecosystem Health Assessment and Its Application in Management: A Multi-Scale Perspective

MEIRONG SU, ZHIFENG YANG, BIN CHEN, GENGYUAN LIU, YAN ZHANG, LIXIAO ZHANG, LINYU XU, AND YANWEI ZHAO

13.1 INTRODUCTION

As a center of production and consumption, urban ecosystems have satisfied human demands throughout most of history. Until recently, the stress of resource depletion and emission of pollutants has remained within the ecosystem's regenerative capacity, and the urban ecosystem was able to self-restore. However, with rapid urbanization, more and more intensive human activities have led to adverse environmental changes that impair societal services and jeopardize sustainability [1]. People have begun to worry about whether the urban ecosystem can support dense populations and provide sustainable services. Therefore, urban ecosystem health has become a scientific topic and a goal of urban development, which integrates the means by which human demands are satisfied with the ecosystem's ability for renewal [2,3].

Owing to its acceptability for managers and the general public, the concept of urban ecosystem health has been extensively applied in practical urban planning and management. Particularly, urban ecosystem health assessments have been widely conducted to comprehensively measure the operations of urban ecosystems, identify limiting factors and provide suggestions for urban management. Accelerated by practical demand, the assessment indicators [4–8] and methods [9–13] have developed quickly on a scientific foundation [14,15].

Reviewing this development, urban ecosystem health assessments are usually conducted on the local scale. In fact, the urban ecosystem is a typical complex open system that links closely with its surroundings through various energy and material flows as well as information circulation. Regarding this intrinsic linkage and influence within urban ecosystem itself and its wider surroundings, the urban ecosystem should be conceptualized at multiple layers. Here, the urban ecosystem plays different roles with different functions. Based on this concept, urban ecosystem health assessments at multiple scales are necessary, which will contribute to a multifaceted understanding of urban ecosystem health status and provide more references for urban management.

In this paper, a novel framework of multi-scale urban ecosystem health assessment and its applications in management are established from the global, national, regional and local scale view points. It is established considering the concerned factors of urban ecosystem health and multi-layer roles of urban ecosystem. Following this, the paper demonstrates an application of the framework using Guangzhou City, China as a case study. The last section offers some discussion and conclusions.

13.2 FACTORS OF CONCERN FOR URBAN ECOSYSTEM HEALTH

Urban ecosystem health is a holistic conception that integrates various factors, such as economic development, social progress, environmental quality, and population health. Meanwhile, it not only emphasizes the current situation but also has a dynamic objective. To understand urban ecosystem health as comprehensively and concisely as possible, we explain it from three dimensions, as shown in Figure 1.

1. The traditional dimension lies on the horizontal axis. The concept of ecosystem health (for natural ecosystems) has developed by only focusing on the characteristics of the ecosystem itself [16] or only on services for humans [17,18]. This has resulted in a combination of characteristics of ecosystems and services for humans [2,3]. Therefore, the concept of urban ecosystem health naturally combines the ability to satisfy reasonable human demands and maintain its own renewal and self-generative capacity since its inception.
2. The stress dimension lies on the eleven-five o'clock axis. A healthy urban ecosystem not only performs well in terms of structural stability and functional completeness under normal conditions, but it also has a strong ability to adapt and recover under serious threat.
3. The temporal dimension lies on the one-seven o'clock axis. Urban ecosystem health regards the growth and development potential for the future as equally important as the current and previous health status, guided by ideas of sustainable development. Attributed to its value-driven characteristics that are strongly influenced by human perceptions [19], urban ecosystem health should be conceptualized as a process [20,21], which can give us much more hope and impel us to focus more studies on the dynamic trends of health status.

13.3 MULTI-LAYER ROLES OF URBAN ECOSYSTEMS

Although urban ecosystem health is described in terms of the three dimensions in Section 2, the focus restricts only on the layer of the urban ecosystem itself. Each system has multiple roles at different layers with different functions [22–24]. Similarly, urban ecosystems can be analyzed from different layers with each analysis helping to understand and provide a special reference to urban ecosystem health from its own viewpoint (see Figure 2).

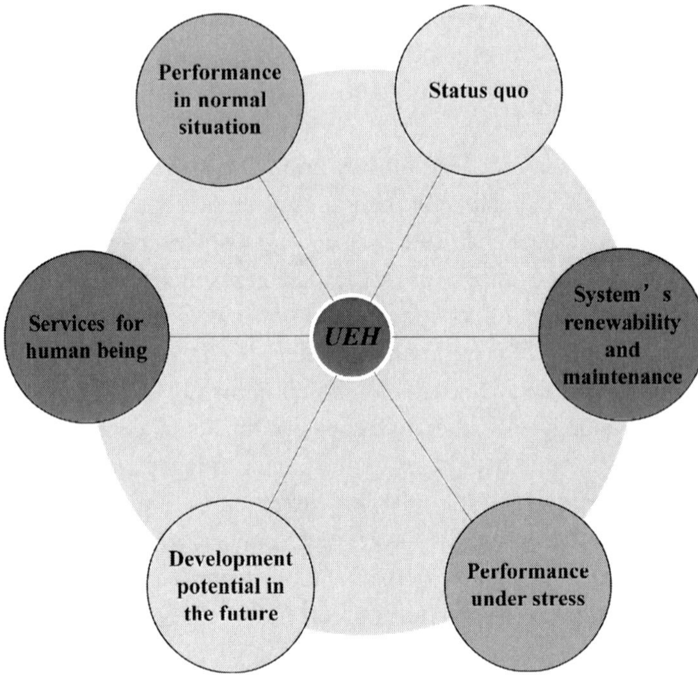

Figure 1. Factors of concern for urb an ecosystem health. (UEH is used in this figure to represent urban ecosystem health).

1. At the local layer, the urban ecosystem itself is a whole system composed of multiple subsystems and various elements. It has its own holistic structure and diverse functions with special characteristics of temporal and spatial change. Urban ecosystem health assessments can verify whether the structure is reasonable, whether different subsystems are harmonious with each other, whether its function is complete, and whether the change in trends is acceptable and sustainable.
2. At the regional layer, different adjacent urban ecosystems interact with each other. Because of the spatial adjacency, they share similar natural conditions and culture, thus there exists an opportunity for both cooperation and completion. Good relationships among different urban ecosystems will bring environmental benefits (e.g.,

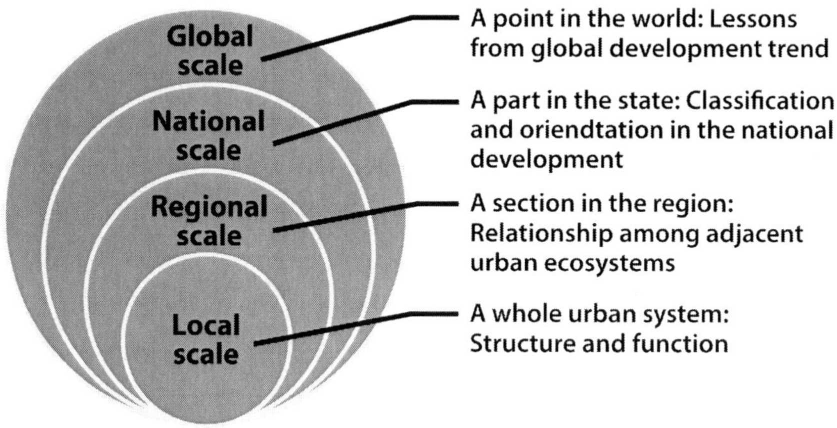

Figure 2. Multi-layer roles of urban ecosystems and respective concerns.

improving resources usage efficiency), which may further lead to improvement of its urban ecosystem health status.

3. At the national layer, different regions or urban ecosystems play different roles according to the national development strategy. The macro-orientation of a concerned urban ecosystem needs to be considered to objectively understand different classifications of urban ecosystem health modes.
4. At the global layer, international development trends and long-term systemic characteristics of human-environment relations influence every urban ecosystem [25]. Valuable experience from urban environmental management and ecological construction can contribute to improvement of the health of concerned urban ecosystems.

13.4 MULTI-SCALE URBAN ECOSYSTEM HEALTH ASSESSMENT AND ITS APPLICATIONS IN MANAGEMENT

Combining the above-mentioned factors of urban ecosystem health and multi-layer roles of urban ecosystems, a novel framework of multi-scale urban ecosystem health assessment applications in management is established, as indicated in Figure 3, which summarizes urban ecosystem health assessment, potential findings of urban ecosystem health assessment, and corresponding contribution for urban management on the global, national, regional and local scales.

Traditionally, the urban ecosystem health assessment is restricted to a local scale, ignoring the multi-layer roles of the urban ecosystem. Here, by analyzing urban ecosystems from multiple scales and applying the multi-scale urban ecosystem health assessment, a more comprehensive viewpoint, more accurate orientation, and more feasible program can guide urban regulation and management. The urban ecosystem health assessment can be conducted in the order of global, national, regional, and local scales, from macro to micro, and rough to detailed analysis. The analysis at larger scales can continuously guide urban management in this way.

13.5 CASE STUDY

Guangzhou, a city located in Guangdong Province, China, helps to illustrate the above framework in more detail. With an area of 7,434.4 km^2, Guangzhou is a modern metropolitan region that supports a population of over 8.0 million (2010 data from [26]). It is the political, economic, and cultural center of Guangdong Province and serves as a commercial, financial, and information center in South China.

As demonstrated above, the urban ecosystem health assessment gradually becomes more detailed and focused at smaller scales. The results of the assessment at the macro-scale shape the rough focus at the micro-scale. At the same time, the results at the micro-scale show concrete decomposed situations and provide more applicable and acceptable suggestions for urban regulation and management.

13.6 DISCUSSION AND CONCLUSIONS

Urban ecosystem is a typical complex open system. It links closely with its surroundings through energy and material flows, information circulation,

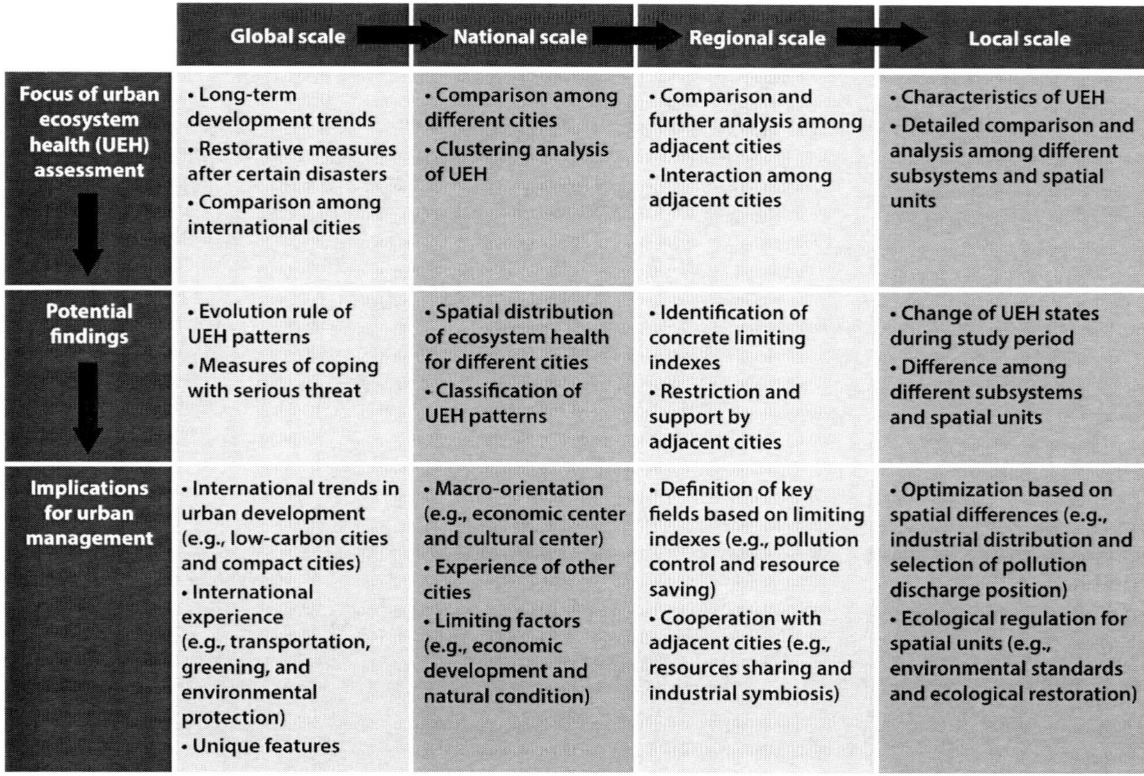

Figure 3. Framework of multi-scale urban ecosystem health assessment and its implications in management.

Table 1. Multi-scale urban ecosystem health assessment for Guangzhou and its implications for management.

Scale	Global scale	National scale
Results of urban ecosystem health assessment	Environmental quality is the main constraint of urban performance, especially as the air quality is low [27].	Guangzhou and other Chinese cities like Beijing, Tianjin, and Shanghai, with relative weak health levels, are classified in the same group.Their common characteristics include high urbanization, high industrialization, and high environmental impacts. The latter is the main restriction of health levels [12].
Implications for management	Measures aiming at creatinga green city, eco-city, compact city, and low-carbon city in international cities are useful reference points. Holistic regulation of land use, public transportation, energy and resource efficiency, and waste treatment need be implemented.	As a regional economic center, various activities arelikely to be intensified, supported by dense energy and flow of resources. Means of using energy and resourcesefficiently should be established to pursue harmony between economic development and environmental protection.
Results of urban ecosystem health assessment	Concrete indicators related to environmental impact are compared for Guangzhou and other cities in the Pearl River Delta. The limiting factors of Guangzhou are identified aslimited local renewable energy sources, small carrying capacity, high dependence on imported energy and resources, and large amounts of waste [28].	The spatial distribution of health levelsin Guangzhou is revealed.The north of Guangzhou is defined as a conservation area, the middle and southern parts are defined as maintenance areas, while the south central and southwestern parts are defined as key regulation areas [29].
Implications for management	In order to slow down the rate of energy depletion and reduce dependence on imports, relevant energy policy and efficient energy usage needs to be proposed [30]. Measures on population control and waste treatment should be strengthened to enlarge the carrying capacity. Cooperation among adjacent cities should be conducted to construct a circular economic chain and realize the optimized cost-benefit budget.	Zoning management should be implemented. Natural resources should be protected and human activities limited in northern parts of the region. Measures to improve economic productivity and energy efficiency, and maintain indigenous renewable resources should be implemented in middle and southern parts of the region. For south central and southwestern parts, more space should be allocated for environmental-friendly production, green consumption patterns should be promoted, energy demands should be reduced, and waste discharge should be reduced.

[a] Non-specific comparison of urban ecosystem health states among Guangzhou and international cities has been done. The results are obtained from comparison among Beijing and international cities.

and cultural communication. The environment undoubtedly has a great impact on urban development. For a given urban ecosystem, the relationship with adjacent cities and the position in the national development scenario will contribute to an objective understanding of its urban ecosystem health status. However, it does not provide insight into the internal situation of the urban ecosystem itself. Therefore, urban ecosystem health assessment at multiple scales is necessary, through which comprehensive suggestions can be given for urban regulation and management.

Considering these demands, a novel framework of multi-scale urban ecosystem health assessment and its applications in management is established. Compared with the traditional urban ecosystem health assessment focusing on the urban ecosystem itself, by integrating situations at global, national, regional, and local scales, the new framework can provide a more comprehensive understanding of urban ecosystem health, more accurate orientation for urban development, and more feasible programs of urban regulation and management. From the macro- to micro-scales, the urban ecosystem health assessment becomes more detailed and focused, and then more applicable and acceptable suggestions can be proposed for urban management.

Only a framework of multi-scale urban ecosystem health assessment and its applications in management are established in this paper, and only the Guangzhou case study is given as a rough demonstration. Further work is required on both the theoretical and practice dimensions to amend the framework. With more applications and sufficient data, the quantitative results of urban ecosystem health assessment at different scales can be further compared, based on which more visible results and valuable references can be obtained for actual management. Because the focus and some indicators of urban ecosystem health assessment may differ with the scale of study, the information integrated needs to be analyzed carefully [31], which can be gradually perfected with more studies.

Urban ecosystem health assessments can provide many valuable references for urban management, including status quo assessment and problem identification, optimization of urban planning and management schemes, and effect evaluation of schemes. However, it should be pointed out that many other disciplines and methods are vital for actual urban management, like system science, landscape ecology, network analysis methods, multi-objective programming methods [32–34], ecological suitability analysis methods, sensitivity analysis methods, and cost-benefit analysis methods.

REFERENCES

1. Vitousek, P.M.; Mooney, H.A.; Lubchenco, J.; Melillo, J.M. Human dominance of Earth's ecosystems. Science 1997, 277, 494–499.
2. O'Laughlin, J. Forest ecosystem health assessment issues: Definition, measurement, and management implications. Ecosyst. Health 1996, 2, 19–39.
3. Rapport, D.J.; Böhm, G.; Buckingham, D.; Cairns, J., Jr.; Costanza, R.; Karr, J.R.; de Kruijf, H.A.M.; Levins, R.; McMichael, A.J.; Nielsen, N.O.; et al. Ecosystem health: The concept, the ISEH, and the important tasks ahead. Ecosyst. Health 1999, 5, 82–90.
4. Harpham, T. Urban health in the Gambia: A review. HealthPlace1996, 2, 45–49.
5. Takano, T.; Nakamura, K. An analysis of health levels and various indicators of urban environments for Healthy Cities projects. J. Epidemiol. Commun. Health 2001, 55, 263–270.
6. Guo, X.R.; Yang, J.R.; Mao, X.Q. Primary studies on urban ecosystem health assessment (in Chinese). China Environ. Sci. 2002, 22, 525–529.
7. Su, M.R.; Yang, Z.F.; Chen, B.;Ulgiati, S. Urban ecosystem health assessment based on emergy and set pair analysis—A comparative study of typical Chinese cities. Ecol. Model 2009, 220, 2341–2348.
8. Spiegel, J.M.; Bonet. M.; Yassi, A.; Molina, E.; Concepcion, M.; Mast, P. Developing ecosystem health indicators in centro Habana: A community-based approach. Ecosyst. Health 2001, 7, 15–26.
9. Zhou, W.H.; Wang, R.S. An entropy weight approach on the fuzzy synthetic assessment of Beijing urban ecosystem health, China (in Chinese). Acta Ecologica. Sinica. 2005, 25, 1344–1351.
10. Yan, W.T. Research on urban ecosystem health attribute synthetic assessment model and application (in Chinese). Syst. Eng. Theor. Practice 2007, 8,137–145.
11. Su, M.R.; Yang, Z.F.; Chen, B. Relative urban ecosystem health assessment: A method integrating comprehensive evaluation and detailed analysis. Ecohealth 2010, 7, 459–472.
12. Liu, G.Y.; Yang, Z.F.; Chen, B.; Ulgiati, S. Emergy-based urban health evaluation and development pattern analysis. Ecol. Model 2009, 220, 2291–2301.
13. Müller, F.; Lenz, R. Ecological indicator: Theoretical fundamentals of consistent applications in environmental management. Ecol. Indic. 2006, 6, 1–5.
14. Costanza, R.; Norton, B.G.; Haskell, B.D. Ecosystem Health: New Goals for Environmental Management, 1st ed.; Island Press: Washington, DC, USA, 1992.

15. Odum, E.P. Perturbation theory and the subsidy-stress gradient. Bioscience 1979, 29, 349–352.
16. Karr, J.R.;Fausch, K.D.; Angermeier, P.L.; Yant, P.R.; Schlosser, I.J. Assessing Biological Integrity in Running Waters: A Method and Its Rationale, 1st ed.; Illinois Natural History Survey: Champaign, State, USA, 1986.
17. Rapport, D.J. What constitute ecosystem health? Perspect. Biol. Med. 1989, 33, 120–132.
18. Mageau, M.T.; Costanza, R.; Ulanowicz, R.E. The development and initial testing of a quantitative assessment of ecosystem health. Ecosyst. Health 1995, 1, 201–213.
19. Odum, E.P. Ecology and Our Endangered Life-support Systems, 1st ed.; Sinauer Associates: Sunderland, State, USA, 1989.
20. Su, M.R.; Fath, B.D.; Yang, Z.F. Urban ecosystem health assessment: A review. Sci. Total Environ. 2010, 408, 2425–2434.
21. Ramalho, C.E.; Hobbs, R.J. Time for a change: Dynamic urban ecology. Trends Ecol. Evol. 2012, 27, 179–188.
22. Brenner, N. Beyond state-centrism? Space, territoriality, and geographical scale in globalization studies. Theor. Soc. 1999, 28, 39–71.
23. Sassen, S.; Dotan, N. Delegating, not returning, to the biosphere: How to use the multi-scalar and ecological properties of cities. Global Environ. Chang. 2011, 21, 823–834.
24. Cai, Y.P.; Huang, G.H.; Tan, Q.; Liu, L. An integrated approach for climate-change impact analysis and adaptation planning under multi-level uncertainties. Part II: Case study. Renew. Sust. Energ. Rev.2011, 15, 3051–3073.
25. Mauro, S.E.D. Seeing the local in the global: Political ecologies, world-systems,and the question of scale. Geoforum 2009, 40, 116–125.
26. Guangzhou Municipal Statistics Bureau. Guangzhou Statistical Yearbook 2011 (in Chinese). Available online: http://data.gzstats.gov.cn/gzStat1/chaxun/njsj.jsp (accessed on 6 November 2012).
27. Wang, J.; Su, M.R.; Chen, B.; Chen, S.Q.; Liang, C. A comparative study of Beijing and three global cities: A perspective on urban livability. Front. Earth Sci. 2011, 5, 323–329.
28. Su, M.R.; Yang, Z.F.; Chen, B. Limiting factor analysis of urban ecosystems based on emergy—A case study of three cities in the Pearl River Delta in China. Procedia. Environ. Sci. 2011, 5, 131–138.
29. Su, M.R.; Fath, B.D. Spatial distribution of urban ecosystem health in Guangzhou, China. Ecol. Indic. 2012, 15, 122–130.
30. Donoso, P.; de Grange, L. A microeconomic interpretation of the maximum entropy estimator of multinomial logit models and its equivalence to the maximum likelihood estimator. Entropy 2010, 12, 2077–2084.
31. Smajgl, A.; House, A.P.N.; Butler, J.R.A. Implications of ecological data constraints for integrated policy and livelihoods modelling: An example from East Kalimantan, Indonesia. Ecol. Model. 2011, 222, 888–896.
32. Cai, Y.P.; Huang, G.H.; Tan, Q. An inexact optimization model for regional energy systems planning in the mixed stochastic and fuzzy environment. Int. J. Energ. Res. 2009, 33, 443–468.

33. Tan, Q.; Huang, G.H.; Cai, Y.P. Waste management with recourse: An inexact dynamic programming model containing fuzzy boundary intervals in objectives and constraints. J. Environ. Manage. 2010, 91, 1898–1913.
34. Tan, Q.; Huang, G.H.; Wu, C.Z.; Cai, Y.P.; Yan, X.P. Development of an inexact fuzzy robust programming model for integrated evacuation management under uncertainty. J. Urban. Plan D ASCE 2009, 135, 39–49.

Author Notes

CHAPTER 4

Acknowledgments

This project was funded by California Energy Commission's Public Interest Energy Research Program under contract 500-10-009. The authors would like to thank Emmanuel Liban and other staff at LA Metro, Alberto Ayala and Shaohua Hu (California Air Resources Board), Paul Bunje (UCLA), Julia Campbell (UCLA and LA Metro), Pierre DuVair (California Energy Commission), and Andrew Fraser (Arizona State University) for their support and input.

CHAPTER 5

Acknowledgements

The authors wish to thank IWT Flanders (Institute for the Promotion of Innovation by Science and Technology in Flanders), FPS Economy (Federal Public Service), Life+ and EFRO (European Union), INTERREG and the Ministry of the Brussels-Capital Region—Brussels Mobility for the (financial) support of the different projects.

Author Contributions

E.L.B and A.B. both coordinated and supervised the different research projects involving photocatalytic applications; E.L.B. prepared the manuscript. All authors read and approved the manuscript.

Conflicts of Interest

The authors declare no conflict of interest.

CHAPTER 6

Acknowledgements

The authors are thankful to the officials at Pradeshiya Sabha, Kaduwela for their immense support in carrying out this project.

CHAPTER 7

Conflicts of Interest

The authors declare no conflict of interest.

CHAPTER 8

Acknowledgments

WATACLIC is a project cofounded by European Commission under the Life+ program. Code of the project is LIFE08 INF/IT/308.

CHAPTER 9

Acknowledgments

This study was supported by Korea Ministry of Environment as The Eco-Innovation project (Global Top project, Project No. GT-SWS-11-01-002-0).

Author Contributions

So-Ryong Chae, Jin-Ho Chung, Yong-Rok Heo, Seok-Tae Kang, and Sang-Min Lee carried out the experiments and wrote the paper; Hang-Sik Shin contributed to the analysis of the experiment data and edited of the manuscript.

Conflicts of Interest

The authors declare no conflict of interest.

CHAPTER 10

Acknowledgments

This work was supported by a grant from the US National Science Foundation IGERT grant (NSF DGE-0654378). We thank ICLEI-USA for facilitating the work with the 20 US cities, the contacts from each of the cities, as well as MIG for providing the IMPLAN data and review of the methods herein.

CHAPTER 11

Acknowledgements

Support for this research was provided by Oak Ridge National Laboratory and the Department of Energy's Office of Policy and International Affairs. We are grateful for the input and guidance provided by the Energy Information Administration, in particular, Erin Boedecker. We would also like to thank Yeong Jae Kim and Paul Baer of the Climate and Energy Policy Laboratory at Georgia Tech for their inputs on the methodology. Lastly, we also wish to thank two anonymous reviewers from Environmental Research Letters for their constructive comments. Any remaining errors in this paper are the responsibility of the authors alone.

CHAPTER 12

Acknowledgements

The authors would like to thank Peter Thomas and Jochen Zeisel from HATI GmbH, Germany, as well as Bernd Genath, Peter Grönewall, and partners of the Terraboga Project for their productive discussion and for sharing their experiences of the German case studies, the Berlin youth center and the Hamburg toilet facility.

This research was, in part, supported by Basic Science Research Program through the National Research Foundation of Korea (NRF) funded by the Ministry of Education, Science and Technology (S-2012-0506-000) and by a grant (11 High-tech Urban G04) from High-tech Urban Development Program funded by Ministry of Land, Transport and Maritime Affairs of Korean government. This work was supported by funding received from the KORANET Joint Call on Green Technologies, www.koranet.eu.

Conflict of Interest

The authors declare no conflict of interest.

CHAPTER 13

Acknowledgements

Financial support is provided by the National Natural Science Foundation of China (No. 40901269), the National Science Foundation for Innovative Research Group (No. 51121003), and the Fundamental Research Funds for the Central Universities. The authors would also thank the help of the editor and the comments of the reviewers, which significantly improved the quality of this paper.

Index

G

H

I

L

M

S

T

U

V

W